AYURVEDIC YOGA LIFESTYLE FOR WINTER

A Brief Guide to Staying Healthy and Happy During the Cold Season. Inspired by Ancient Wisdom.

Sharmila Panikkal

Ayurvedic yoga lifestyle for winter

CONTENTS

Ayurvedic yoga lifestyle for winter

Ayurvedic yoga lifestyle for winter

PREFACE

Winter, a season that presents unique challenges for both the body and mind, is the focus of this book. It invites you to adopt an Ayurvedic Yoga lifestyle tailored to this transformative time of year.

Yoga is more than just a fitness routine or a profound philosophy; it is a holistic approach to living in harmony with nature and us. In this book, I explore the profound connection between Ayurveda and Yoga, and how their combined wisdom can help you maintain health, fitness, and balance during winter.

Winter often brings seasonal challenges such as the blues, joint discomfort, allergies, asthma, and other health concerns. This guide offers practical and effective solutions for overcoming these difficulties while nurturing your physical, mental, and spiritual well-being. You will discover the Ayurvedic perspective on winter, the relationship between the five elements and the body, and how to make thoughtful lifestyle adjustments to support your overall health.

In addition, this book presents a fitness program specifically designed for winter, aimed at nurturing your mind, body, and spirit. Understanding and applying these principles

Ayurvedic yoga lifestyle for winter

allows you to transform winter into a season of strength, rejuvenation, and growth.

Let this book inspire you to embrace winter fully, enjoy its beauty, and thrive in its challenges. It is not just a book but an invitation to join a community of individuals ready to embrace winter in a new and fulfilling way.

Ayurvedic yoga lifestyle for winter

AYURVEDA AND YOGA SECRETS FOR WINTER

Yoga is the sister science of Ayurveda, and together, they offer profound insights for navigating winter with balance and vitality.

The convergence of Ayurveda and Yoga offers a sophisticated, time-tested framework for maintaining physiological balance and mental clarity during winter. Rooted in ancient Indian philosophy, both disciplines emphasise alignment with natural rhythms, advocating seasonal routines that nurture resilience and vitality.

 Winter, characterised by cold, dryness, and increased kapha dosha, presents unique challenges to the body's homeostasis. Ayurveda recommends tailored dietary modifications and lifestyle. Yoga complements these practices through asanas and pranayama, which are designed to generate internal heat, enhance circulation, and reduce lethargy. These postures are beneficial for energising the body and maintaining muscular flexibility. The respiratory system can be invigorated, nasal passages can be cleared, and pranic energy can

Ayurvedic yoga lifestyle for winter

be awakened during colder months through breathing techniques. Together, Ayurveda and Yoga provide a dual-layered approach, preventive and therapeutic. While Ayurveda focuses on individualised constitution (prakriti) and its interaction with seasonal influences, Yoga fosters internal balance through mindful movement and breath control. Their integration is particularly effective in winter, which often induces sluggishness, compromised immunity, and emotional inertia.

The insights derived from this synthesis encourage an adaptive and intentional lifestyle. Regular practice strengthens the immune system and supports emotional well-being, cognitive function, and spiritual growth. As modern science continues to validate many of the principles espoused by these ancient systems, their relevance and application in today's world become increasingly evident. Through conscious living, guided by Ayurvedic routines and yogic discipline, winter transforms from a season of dormancy into one of deep nourishment and renewal.

Uncover the secrets revealed in this guide if you're ready to embrace winter in the most authentic and fulfilling way! The complementary nature of Ayurveda and yoga makes these two ancient Indian sciences one of

Ayurvedic yoga lifestyle for winter

the best forms of holistic well-being, and there are many ways in which they are inseparable.

Ayurvedic yoga lifestyle for winter

THE TIMELESS PRINCIPLES OF AYURVEDA AND YOGA

Welcome to a journey of rediscovering wellness through the timeless principles of Ayurveda and Yoga, specifically tailored for the winter season. These two ancient sciences, deeply rooted in India's cultural and spiritual heritage, are more than just practices; they are a way of life designed to align the body, mind, and spirit with the rhythms of nature.

My roots lie in Kerala, where Ayurveda is not just an alternative system but a way of life. Growing up in an Ayurvedic family, I witnessed the profound impact of holistic living and natural remedies. My grandfather, a respected Ayurvedic practitioner, healed countless individuals by guiding them towards a balanced lifestyle. His work was a living testament to the power of harmony, balance, and mindfulness.

In Kerala, many still consider Ayurvedic doctors their first point of contact for health concerns, with modern medicine often called "English medicine." This distinction reflects not just a cultural mindset but a preference for natural, integrative approaches to healing. This

Ayurvedic yoga lifestyle for winter

preference is gaining momentum and uniting people globally, including you, the reader of this book.

However, much of its holistic essence was lost when Yoga travelled to the West. Stripped of its Ayurvedic context, Yoga became seen primarily as a physical fitness program, overlooking its more profound purpose of fostering balance and wellness. Thankfully, this narrative is changing, and more people are embracing Ayurveda and Yoga together, offering a hopeful and exciting future for a powerful holistic healing system. This future is one where balance and wellness are ideals and achievable realities for all who commit to this lifestyle.

This book is not just a collection of information but an invitation to explore Ayurvedic Yoga as a lifestyle for winter. This season often challenges our physical and mental resilience. By understanding your unique constitution, or dosha, and adjusting your routines, diet, and Yoga practice to suit the season, you can create a lifestyle that actively supports your well-being through the colder months.

Embark on a journey of self-discovery and wellness with this book. Learn how to align your body, mind, and spirit with the rhythms of

Ayurvedic yoga lifestyle for winter

nature through the timeless principles of Ayurveda and Yoga.

This book consists of sixteen chapters, thoughtfully and explicitly crafted for the winter season.

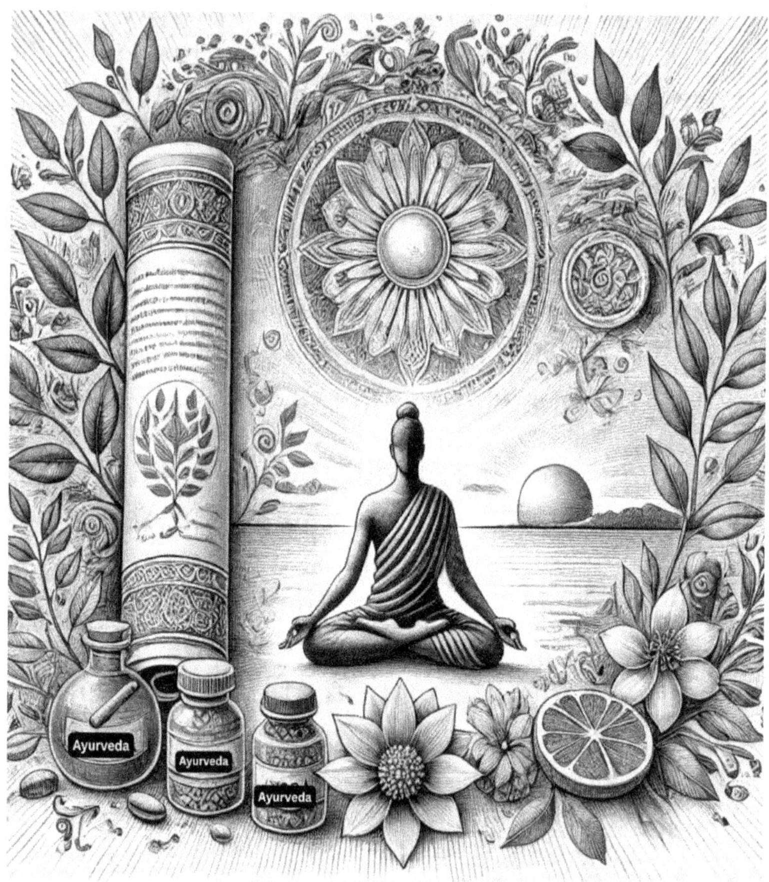

Discover the transformative path to mindful living through the integration of timeless principles from Ayurveda and Yoga. With this

Ayurvedic yoga lifestyle for winter

guide, you will unlock the potential to turn winter into a season of deep rest, refreshing rejuvenation, and vibrant holistic health.

Let this book be your trusted companion for thriving during the colder months, making this winter a time of growth, balance, and harmony for your mind, body, and spirit.

This simple yet profound idea reminds us that our experience of the environment largely depends on how well we prepare for it. Just as the right layers of clothing can turn a harsh winter day into a pleasant experience, adopting the proper lifestyle and daily habits can help us thrive, regardless of the season.

Ayurvedic yoga lifestyle for winter

A BRIEF GUIDE FOR WINTER

Winter can present various physical obstacles, but we can fully appreciate its beauty by caring for our body, mind, and spirit in harmony with the season. Ayurveda states that the weather significantly influences our overall well-being, affecting the mind, body, and spirit. By adhering to Ayurvedic principles, it is possible to survive and thrive during winter. It's important to grasp the influence of the three doshas and the five elements during different seasons. These seasonal influences can have a profound impact on our health and well-being. Understanding this connection is the key to preventing potential health issues and empowering us to take control of our wellness.
As the Swiss saying goes, "There is no such thing as bad weather, only inappropriate clothing."

 This simple yet profound idea reminds us that our experience of the environment largely depends on how well we prepare for it

Just as the right layers of clothing can turn a harsh winter day into a pleasant experience, adopting the proper lifestyle and daily habits can help us thrive, regardless of the season.

Ayurvedic yoga lifestyle for winter

This principle is deeply embedded in Ayurveda. It teaches that by aligning our routines, diets, and self-care practices with the changing seasons, we can maintain balance and prevent discomfort or disease. Rather than resisting nature, Ayurveda encourages us to adapt intelligently through seasonal foods, warm and grounding practices, and mindful living.

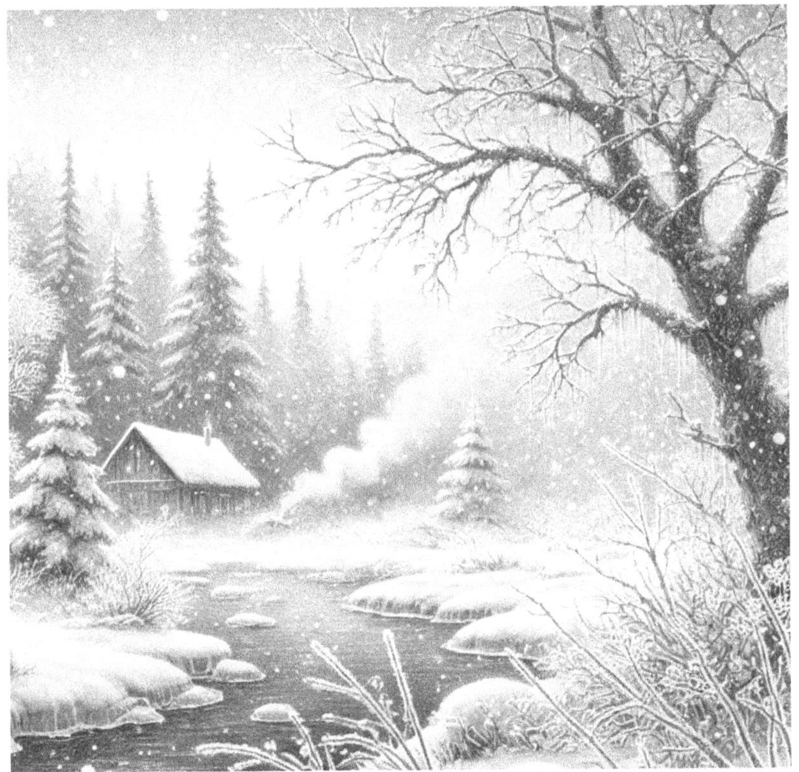

An extreme winter

Ayurvedic yoga lifestyle for winter

This proactive approach transforms winter from a season of struggle into one of strength, warmth, and renewal.

This simple yet profound idea reminds us that our experience of the environment largely depends on how well we prepare for it. Just as the right layers of clothing can turn a harsh winter day into a pleasant experience, adopting the proper lifestyle and daily habits can help us thrive, regardless of the season

Ayurvedic yoga lifestyle for winter

WHAT IS WINTER IN AYURVEDA

In Ayurveda, winter is viewed as a season dominated primarily by the **Kapha dosha**, with **Vata** playing a significant role during the early, transitional phase. The environment during this time mirrors the qualities of these doshas, **cold, heavy, moist, and slow,** all of which influence both the physical and mental state of an individual. According to Ayurvedic wisdom, the body naturally strengthens during winter. The cooler temperatures help **preserve internal heat**, allowing the **digestive fire (Agni)** to burn brighter. This is why people often feel hungrier and can digest heavier foods more efficiently in winter.

Nature, too, undergoes a transformation during this season. Trees shed their leaves, animals retreat into hibernation, and the earth becomes still and quiet. These changes reflect **Kapha's qualities of inertia, stability, and density.** The

Ayurvedic yoga lifestyle for winter

atmosphere becomes dense with moisture, particularly in late winter, increasing the likelihood of congestion, sluggishness, or water retention in the body. At the same time, early winter, with its chill and dryness, can **provoke Vata**, which governs movement, circulation, and nervous system activity. When imbalanced, this may lead to **dry skin, anxiety, insomnia, or joint stiffness**.

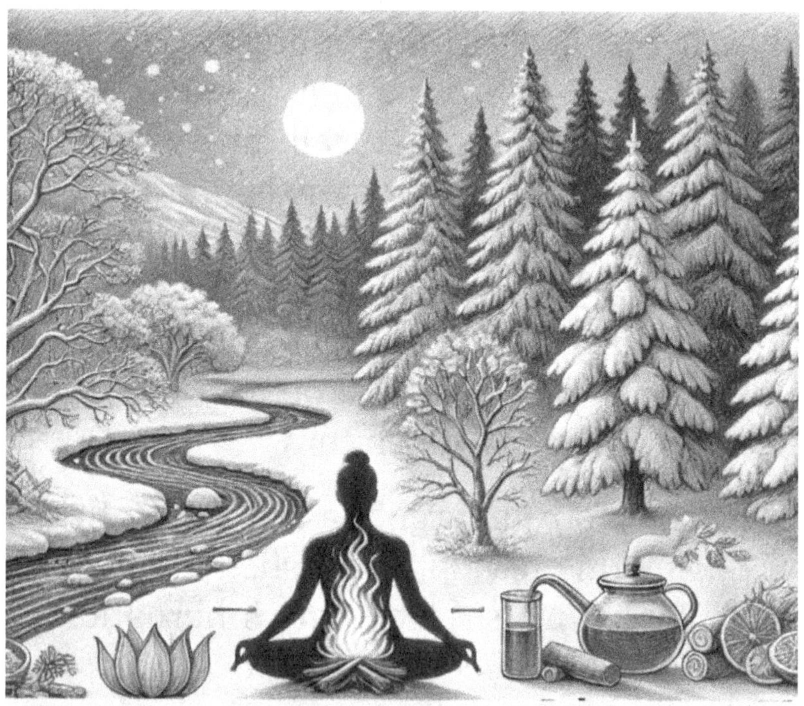

A season primarily influenced by Kapha with a subtle presence of Vata.

Ayurvedic yoga lifestyle for winter

Ayurveda teaches us to recognise these shifts in nature as cues for self-care. By incorporating warm, oily, and grounding foods, staying physically

active, and establishing a consistent daily rhythm, one can maintain equilibrium throughout the season. Self-massage with warm oil, steam therapies, and calming practices such as meditation are also encouraged to counteract the cold and dampness of winter.

Overall, winter in Ayurveda is not just a time of rest, but a powerful opportunity to **strengthen immunity, stabilise the mind, and restore vitality**, if one aligns lifestyle choices with nature's pace and rhythm.

Ayurvedic yoga lifestyle for winter

WHAT IS AYURVEDA

Ayurveda is an ancient system of holistic medicine that originated in India over 5,000 years ago. The word "Ayurveda" comes from the Sanskrit terms "Ayur" (life) and "Veda" (science or knowledge), meaning "the science of life." It emphasizes achieving balance and harmony within the body, mind, and spirit to promote health and prevent illness.

Key principles of Ayurveda include:

- Five Elements (Panchamahabhutas): The universe and the human body are composed of five elements, earth, water, fire, air, and ether (space).
- Doshas: The body is governed by three biological energies or doshas: Vata (air and space), Pitta (fire and water), and Kapha (earth and water).
- Each person has a unique combination of these doshas, which determines their constitution or Prakriti.

Holistic approach: Ayurveda considers diet, lifestyle, mental health, and environmental factors in diagnosing and treating health concerns.

Ayurvedic yoga lifestyle for winter

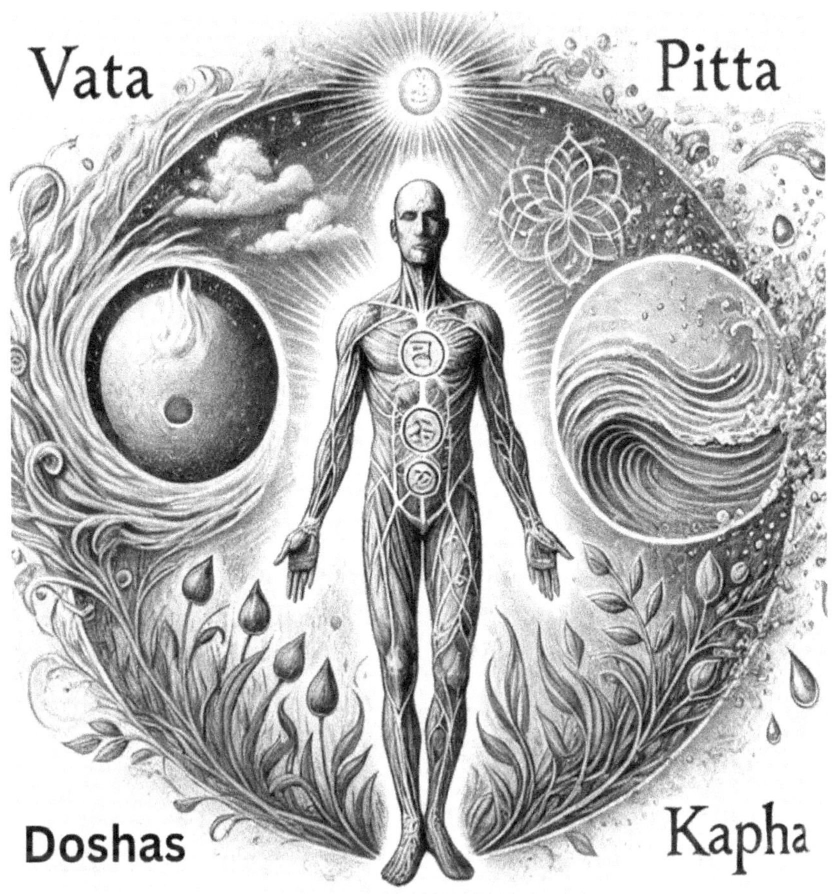

Three Doshas

Ayurveda restores balance using herbs, oils, massage, meditation, yoga, and dietary adjustments. It also focuses on seasonal changes, daily routines (Dinacharya), and, most importantly, individualised treatment plans. This personalised approach ensures that each person's unique constitution and health

Ayurvedic yoga lifestyle for winter

concerns are considered, making them feel valued and unique.

 The goal is to achieve optimal well-being by aligning with nature and fostering self-awareness.

The unique *Prakriti* (natural constitution) of an individual is shaped by the five elements, which govern physical, mental, and emotional traits. *Prakriti* is determined by a specific combination of the three doshas, typically with one being dominant. This results in three primary body types: **Vata-dominant**, **Pitta-dominant**, and **Kapha-dominant**. Each type displays distinct characteristics, behaviours, and preferences. Understanding these traits helps in identifying a person's unique personality.

Recognising your dominant dosha offers valuable understanding of your body's natural rhythms and tendencies. It explains not only physical features and metabolic patterns but also emotional responses, mental clarity, and behavioural inclinations. By becoming aware of your Ayurvedic constitution, you can make informed choices in your daily life, ranging from dietary habits to lifestyle practices, which support internal balance and long-term well-being.

Ayurvedic yoga lifestyle for winter

If you want to explore dosha-specific personalities in greater detail, our guidebook provides practical tools to help you identify and care for your individual constitution. In the next chapter, we will delve further into each body type, enabling you to discover your personal dosha and begin shaping a lifestyle that aligns with your true nature.

Ayurvedic yoga lifestyle for winter

AYURVEDIC PERSONALITY MATTERS

The human body type changes according to its Prakriti (natural constitution) and the balance of the three Doshas—Vata, Pitta, and Kapha. These Doshas are the fundamental life forces in Ayurveda and are governed by the five elements: space, air, fire, water, and earth. The Prakriti of an individual is determined by their unique combination of these elements, which shape their physical, mental, and emotional traits.

The balance between Vata, Pitta, and Kapha is crucial for maintaining harmony in the body and mind. Each person's Prakriti is typically dominated by one Dosha, resulting in three primary body types.

Vata-Dominant: Influenced by space and air, Vata types are light, quick, and flexible.

Pitta-Dominant: Governed by fire and water, Pitta types are dynamic, intense, and ambitious.

Kapha-Dominant: Rooted in earth and water, Kapha types are steady, nurturing, and composed.

Ayurvedic yoga lifestyle for winter

The Importance of Lifestyle and Diet

Understanding one's Prakriti is essential for aligning lifestyle choices, including food, with the body and mind's needs. A balanced diet tailored to the Dosha helps maintain harmony and prevents imbalances.

Imbalances and Their Impacts. Each body type exhibits unique characteristics, behaviours, tendencies, and specific vulnerabilities to imbalance.

For instance, Vata imbalance may cause anxiety, dryness, or restlessness.

Pitta imbalance can lead to anger, inflammation, or overheating.

Kapha imbalance might result in sluggishness, weight gain, or congestion.

One can cultivate balance and enhance well-being by understanding Prakriti, Doshas and lifestyle interplay

How to Identify Your Ayurvedic Personality (Prakriti)?

Your Ayurvedic Personality: Understanding Your Unique Nature

Your *Prakriti* (natural constitution) is formed at birth based on the predominance of the three doshas: **Vata**, **Pitta**, and **Kapha**. Every person has a distinct combination of these energies, with one often being more influential than the

Ayurvedic yoga lifestyle for winter

others. Knowing your constitution allows for smarter lifestyle, diet, and self-care decisions that support your overall well-being.

Why Understanding Your Ayurvedic Personality Matters

Your dosha acts like your internal blueprint, revealing how your body functions, how your mind processes information, and how your emotions flow. This understanding can bring transformative clarity to your health, relationships, and career path.

Relationships: Building Awareness and Connection

Learning about doshas improves how we relate to others:

- **Enhances communication** – For instance, a Pitta may speak directly, while a Kapha prefers gentle, reassuring dialogue.

- **Supports mutual growth** – Vata's spontaneity may balance Kapha's steadiness if there's awareness and respect.

- **Reduces misunderstandings** – Pitta might grow impatient with slower-paced people, while Vata may feel overwhelmed

Ayurvedic yoga lifestyle for winter

by intensity. Recognizing these tendencies helps diffuse potential conflict.

Example: A Vata individual may crave variety and excitement, whereas a Kapha partner may prefer consistency and calm. Knowing these traits fosters compassion and emotional understanding.

Health: Personalized Wellness

Each dosha has its own tendencies:

- **Vata**: Prone to anxiety, dryness, digestive irregularities.

- **Pitta**: Susceptible to inflammation, irritability, and overexertion.

- **Kapha**: May struggle with sluggishness, congestion, and weight gain.

Knowing your dosha helps you:

- Choose foods that maintain internal harmony.

- Pick exercises that suit your energy patterns.

- Establish routines that support emotional and physical vitality.

Example: A Pitta type benefits more from cooling activities like swimming or moonlight

Ayurvedic yoga lifestyle for winter

walks rather than high-heat workouts, which could lead to burnout.

This insight also aids in preventing disease by adjusting habits before imbalance sets in. It improves emotional resilience and strengthens immunity, energy, and digestion naturally.

Career: Working in Alignment with Your Nature

Different doshas flourish in different environments:

- **Vata** thrives in creative roles—design, writing, innovation.

- **Pitta** excels in leadership, technology, law, and strategic thinking.

- **Kapha** is drawn to nurturing roles— teaching, counselling, healthcare.

Understanding your type helps you:

- Choose a work style that suits your natural rhythm.

- Avoid exhaustion by honouring your limits.

- Improve collaboration by appreciating others' working styles.

Ayurvedic yoga lifestyle for winter

Example: A Vata may feel stifled in rigid structures but shine in freelance or artistic roles, while a Kapha may feel at ease in steady, predictable work environments.

In Summary

Knowing your Ayurvedic constitution empowers you to:

- Make better health and nutrition decisions.

- Improve emotional intelligence in personal and professional relationships.

- Select a career path that energizes rather than drains you.

It is not just traditional wisdom; it is a personal guide to navigating life with awareness and balance.

Use the Ayurvedic personality test in this chapter to discover your dosha. Once identified, you can make intentional choices about your routines, diet, and habits to support your physical and mental well-being. This awareness helps reduce stress, promote restful sleep, and keep your energy stable.

Even more, understanding the doshas of your loved ones enhances your ability to relate to

Ayurvedic yoga lifestyle for winter

them with empathy and patience. You will be able to respond to their needs more effectively and reduce unnecessary conflict.

Everything in nature is designed with uniqueness. Although people may appear similar on the surface, each one is distinct at the core. Ayurveda encourages us to embrace this diversity instead of conforming to a single standard of appearance or behaviour.

Take a moment to observe the illustration in this chapter. It highlights how everybody's shape and constitution is a unique creation of nature. Just like a garden full of diverse flowers, the variety of human bodies is a testament to nature's beauty. Attempting to force everyone into a single mould goes against this natural intelligence. Ayurveda invites you to celebrate your individuality and care for yourself with love and respect.

The visual representation shows the three primary Ayurvedic constitutions, Vata, Pitta, and Kapha—each formed through different combinations of the five great elements (*Panchamahabhutas*), and each shaping particular physical, emotional, and mental attributes.

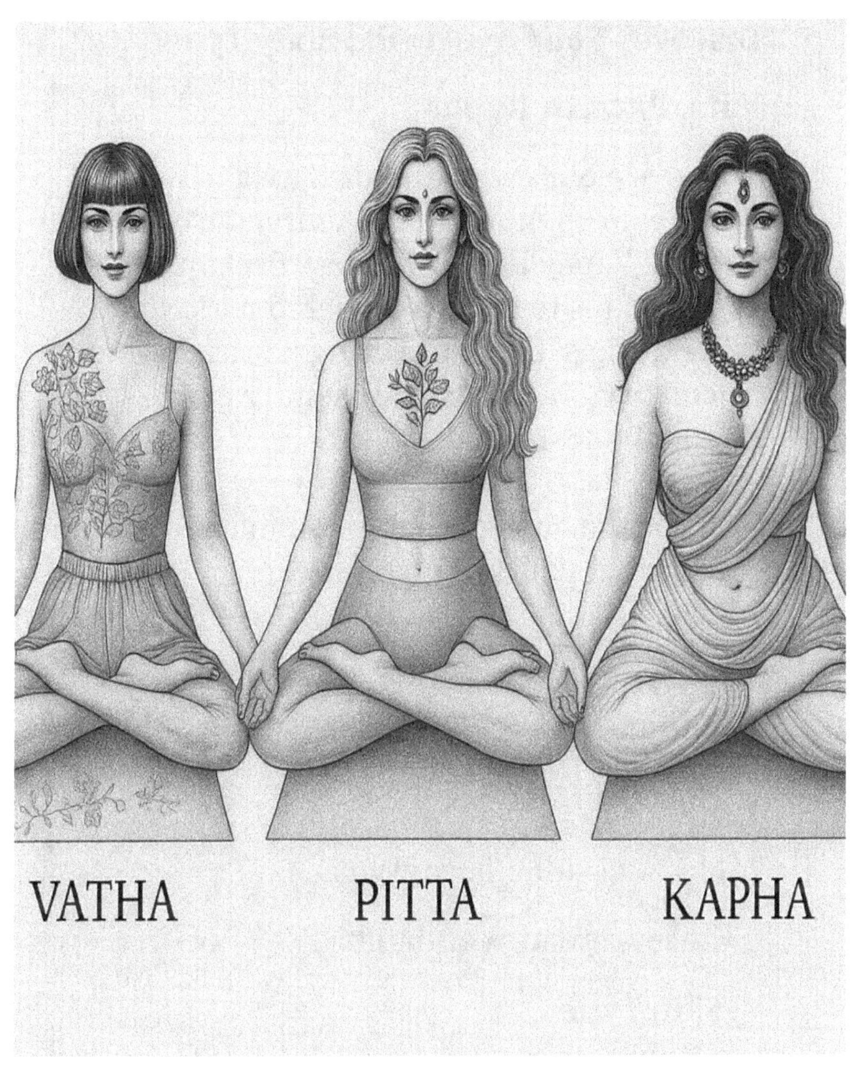

The illustration depicts the three primary
Ayurvedic body and personality types: doshas
Vata, Pitta, and Kapha

Ayurvedic yoga lifestyle for winter

Discover Your Ayurvedic Body Type:

Vata, Pitta, or Kapha

Below is a questionnaire designed to help determine an individual's Ayurvedic body type (Dosha: Vata, Pitta, or Kapha). Each question corresponds to traits associated with the three doshas. Use the scoring key at the end to calculate your points and identify your dominant dosha and Prakriti.

Just tick the answer that is suitable for you, and please do it yourself for this test.

I. Physical Traits

1. Body frame and build

a. Thin, light, and bony

b. Medium, athletic, muscular

c. Stocky, broad, well-built

2. Skin Type

a. Dry, rough, and cool

b. Oily, warm, prone to redness or acne

c. Soft, thick, and moist

3. Hair Type

Ayurvedic yoga lifestyle for winter

a. Thin, dry, frizzy, and brittle

b. Delicate, oily, and prone to early greying

c. Thick, lustrous, and wavy

4. Eye Size and Appearance

a. Small, dry, dull, or restless

b. Medium-sized, sharp, and intense

c. Large, calm, and attractive

5. Hunger and Appetite

a. Irregular appetite, prone to skipping meals

b. Strong appetite, can't skip meals

c. Slow appetite, prefers fewer meals

6. Digestion

a. Irregular, prone to bloating and
   constipation

b. Strong but sensitive, prone to acidity or
   heartburn

c. Slow, heavy, but steady digestion

7. Body Temperature

a. Cold hands and feet, dislikes cold weather

Ayurvedic yoga lifestyle for winter

b. Warm body, dislikes heat and humidity

c. Tolerates cold but dislikes damp or humid weather

8. Weight

a. Difficulty gaining weight

b. Gains and loses weight easily

c. Tends to gain weight and finds it hard to lose

9. Sleep Pattern

a. Light, interrupted sleep

b. Moderate sleep with vivid dreams

c. Deep, heavy sleep, hard to wake up

10. Energy Levels

a. Erratic energy, bursts followed by fatigue

b. steady, moderate stamina

c. Slow but long-lasting energy

II. Mental Characteristics

1. Learning Speed

a. Quick learning but forgetting easily

Ayurvedic yoga lifestyle for winter

b. Sharp and focused learner

c. Learns slowly but remembers well

2. Thinking Process

a. Imaginative, creative, but scattered

b. Logical, analytical, sharp

c. Calm, steady, and methodical

3. Concentration

a. Easily distracted, mind wanders

b. Intense focus on tasks

c. Consistent but slow

4. Decision Making

a. Indecisive, changes mind frequently

b. Quick and confident decisions

c. Takes time to decide but stays firm

5. Problem-Solving Approach

a. Look for creative or unconventional
   solutions

b. Uses logic and rationality

c. Prefers tried-and-tested methods

Ayurvedic yoga lifestyle for winter

6. Memory

a. Quick memory but forgetful

b. Sharp memory, remembering details

c. Long-term memory retains information
   Well,

7. Thought Speed

a. Rapid, racing thoughts

b. Focused and intense thoughts

c. Slow, steady, and deliberate thinking

8. Curiosity

a. Highly curious, enjoys variety

b. Curious about specific interests, deep focus

c. Curious but passive, like familiar topics

9. Imagination

a. Highly imaginative and creative

b. Moderate imagination, preferring realistic
   ideas

c. Low imagination, grounded and practical

10. Speech

Ayurvedic yoga lifestyle for winter

a. Talks quickly, changes topics often

b. Direct, confident, sometimes sharp

c. Slow, measured, and calm

III. Emotional Characteristics

1. Response to Stress

a. Nervous, anxious, or panicked

b. Irritated or angry

c. Calm and composed under stress

2. Emotional Stability

a. Emotional heights and lows, unpredictable

b. Passionate, sometimes volatile

c. Stable, slow to react emotionally

3. Anger

a. Rarely angry but feels nervous instead

b. Easily angered but calms down quickly

c. Rarely angry but holds onto resentment

4. Fear

a. Prone to fear and worry

b. Fearless, bold, confrontational

Ayurvedic yoga lifestyle for winter

c. Calm and rarely fearful

5. Compassion

a. Compassionate but inconsistent

b. Empathetic but goal-focused

c. Deeply nurturing and compassionate

6. Excitement

a. Easily excited, enthusiastic

b. Controlled excitement, goal-oriented

c. Calm and not easily excited

7. Forgiveness

a. Forgives easily but forgets lessons

b. Forgives but may hold grudges

c. Forgives easily and rarely holds grudges

8. Patience

a. Impatient, restless

b. Moderately patient, focused

c. Very patient, easy-going

9. Sensitivity

a. Highly sensitive, overreacts

Ayurvedic yoga lifestyle for winter

b. Sensitive but practical

c. Low sensitivity remains grounded

10. Social Interaction

a. Social, enjoys a variety of interactions

b. Prefers meaningful, focused
   interactions

c. Prefers close, long-term relationships

IV. Lifestyle Characteristics

1. Work Style

a. Starts projects enthusiastically but
   struggles to finish

b. Goal-oriented, thrives under
   pressure

c. Consistent, prefer steady, routine
   work

2. Activity Levels

a. Restless, likes to move constantly

b. Likes competitive activities

c. Slow and steady, prefers relaxed

Ayurvedic yoga lifestyle for winter

activities

3. Dietary Preferences

a. Light, dry, crunchy foods

b. Spicy, sour, salty Flavors

c. Sweet, heavy, and oily foods

4. Exercise Preference

a. Light activities like yoga or walking

b. Intense workouts, running, or

   competitive sports

c. Gentle, low-intensity exercises like

swimming

5. Sleep Pattern

a. Light, interrupted sleep

b. Moderate sleep with vivid dreams

c. Deep, heavy, uninterrupted sleep

6. Response to Routine

a. Dislikes routine, prefers variety

b. Prefers a structured and efficient

   routine

Ayurvedic yoga lifestyle for winter

c. Thrives on consistency and routine

7. Reaction to Weather

a. Dislikes cold, dry weather

b. Dislikes hot, humid weather

c. Dislikes cold, damp weather

8. Craving for Food

a. Craves salty or crunchy snacks

b. Craves spicy or tangy foods

c. Craving, creamy, or rich foods

9. Spending Habits

an Impulsive, spends on whims

b. Strategic and purposeful spending

c. conservative, cautious with money

10. Interaction with Others

a. social butterfly, loves meeting new people

b. Focused on meaningful connections

c. Prefers close-knit, long-term relationships

Ayurvedic yoga lifestyle for winter

Scoring and Interpretation

Assign: 1 point for each Vata (a), Pitta (b), Kapha (c) response. Tally the total for each dosha out of 40. The dosha with the highest score reflects your dominant Prakriti,

When calculating the score

If one dosha scores the highest, it is considered your dominant dosha. If two doshas have equal or nearly equal scores, it is considered a dual dosha constitution (e.g., Vata-Pitta, Pitta-Kapha, or Vata-Kapha).
If all three doshas score equally or nearly equally, it is considered Samadosha, meaning a balanced constitution where Vata, Pitta, and Kapha are in harmony.

Why Dosha Balance is Important

Even though you have a dominant dosha, you can still experience imbalances in other doshas due to age, season, and weather. According to Ayurveda, human life is divided into different stages, each governed by a specific dosha - Vata, Pitta, or Kapha.
These doshas influence not only physical health but also mental and emotional well-being. Ayurveda's chronological age with dosha dominance helps us understand how our bodies change over time.

Ayurvedic yoga lifestyle for winter

Like age, seasons also influence our doshas, affecting our bodies, minds, and health. Understanding the seasonal impact of doshas helps us adjust our lifestyle and diet to maintain balance.

The Impact of Seasonal Changes on Dosha Balance

Dominant dosha governs each season, and if your body type, age, and seasonal alien With the same dosha, you may experience increased imbalance. For example, Autumn and early Winter are known as the Vata Season because they are dry, cold, and windy. Dominant Dosha: Vata (Air & Ether elements), Season-Late fall to early winter (October to February, depending on the climate), which can create Increased dryness in the skin, hair, and joints. Fluctuating energy levels. Anxiety, restlessness, Irregular digestion, bloating, or constipation. In this situation, Vata-dominant people above 50 years old and living in the Vata season (autumn or early winter) are more prone to Vata-related imbalances. If they do not maintain balance through the proper diet and lifestyle, they may face joint issues, anxiety, poor digestion, and dryness. At the same time, while one dosha dominates a particular phase of life or season, imbalances can still occur in

Ayurvedic yoga lifestyle for winter

the other doshas if lifestyle choices are not aligned properly.

For example, A person in the Kapha phase of life (0-16 years) or living in the Kapha season (late winter/spring) can develop excess Kapha imbalances, like weight gain or mucus buildup, if they follow a heavy, sluggish lifestyle. Similarly, a person in their Pitta phase (16-50 years) or in the Pitta season (summer) can experience excess heat, inflammation, and digestive issues if they do not follow a cooling diet and lifestyle.

Ayurveda teaches that understanding your personal dosha, age, and seasonal influences allows you to make conscious lifestyle adjustments. Please check the characteristics of each dosha below by eating the right foods, following the proper routines, and being mindful of seasonal shifts. Understanding these traits will help you recognise different personality types, allowing you to make more informed choices when selecting a career, partner, or relationship. Aligning with the right dosha type can bring greater harmony to your life on all levels.

In Ayurveda, there is no single general rule; each of us is a unique universe creation. By

Ayurvedic yoga lifestyle for winter

identifying your uniqueness, you can embrace and celebrate your life fully.

Doshas, characteristics, and personality.
1. Vata Dosha
Element: Air and Ether (Space)
Qualities: Dry, light, cold, rough, mobile, subtle
Physical
Characteristics Body Frame: Thin, light, often underweight, with prominent joints and veins.
Skin: Dry, rough, cool, prone to cracking and sensitivity.
Hair: Thin, dry, frizzy, prone to breakage or split ends.
Eyes: Small, dull, or restless, with a tendency to dryness.
Appetite: Irregular, variable hunger.
Digestion: Prone to bloating, gas, and constipation.
Sleep: Light, disturbed sleep; prone to insomnia.
Energy: Erratic bursts of energy, followed by fatigue.

Mental Characteristics
Thinking: Creative, imaginative, but scattered.
Memory: Quick to grasp new ideas but forgets easily.
Decision-Making: Indecisive, changes mind frequently.

Ayurvedic yoga lifestyle for winter

Focus: Struggles with prolonged focus.

Emotional Characteristics
Response to Stress: Nervousness, anxiety, fear.
Emotions: Tends to worry or overthink.
Social Nature: Enjoys variety and new experiences but gets easily overwhelmed.

2. Pitta Dosha
Element: Fire and Water
Qualities: Hot, sharp, oily, intense, light Physical Characteristics
Body Frame: Medium build, muscular, with moderate weight.
Skin: Warm, oily, prone to redness, rashes, or acne. Hair: Fine, straight, oily, prone to early greying or thinning.
Eyes: Medium-sized, sharp, intense gaze.
Appetite: Strong, can't skip meals.
Digestion: Strong but sensitive; prone to acidity or heartburn.
Sleep: Moderate sleep; dreams are often vivid.
Energy: Consistent and high energy levels, but easily exhausted.

Mental Characteristics
Thinking: Logical, analytical, sharp intellect.
Memory: Excellent memory; quick to recall details.
Decision-Making: Confident and decisive.

Ayurvedic yoga lifestyle for winter

Focus: Intense and goal-oriented.

Emotional Characteristics

Response to Stress: Irritability, frustration, anger.
Emotions: Passionate and competitive but may struggle with temper. Social Nature:
Prefers meaningful, focused interactions.

3. Kapha Dosha

Element: Earth and Water
Qualities: Heavy, slow, steady, cool, moist
Physical Characteristics
Body Frame: Large, stocky, broad build; gains weight easily.
Skin: Thick, soft, cool to touch, and moist.
Hair: Thick, lustrous, wavy, and oily. Eyes:
Large, calm, attractive, often moist.
Appetite: Slow but steady.
Digestion: Sluggish, prone to heaviness or indigestion.
Sleep: Deep, heavy sleep; hard to wake up.
Energy: Slow to start but sustains energy for a long time.

Mental Characteristics

Thinking: Steady, methodical, and thoughtful.
Memory: Slow to grasp new ideas, but excellent long-term retention.

Ayurvedic yoga lifestyle for winter

Decision-Making: Takes time to decide but rarely changes decisions.
Focus: Strong but slow-moving.

Emotional Characteristics
Response to Stress: Calm, steady, avoids confrontation.
Emotions: Nurturing, compassionate, forgiving.
Social Nature: Prefers close, long-term relationships.

4. Dual Doshas
Many individuals exhibit characteristics of two dominant doshas rather
than one.
Vata-Pitta Characteristics
Physical: Thin build (Vata), warm skin (Pitta), prone to dryness and sensitivity.
Mental: Creative and analytical, with scattered but focused thoughts when balanced.
Emotional: Tends to worry (Vata) but can also show irritability

(Pitta). Pitta-Kapha
Physical Characteristics: Medium-to-large build, strong and steady energy. Mental: Sharp intellect (Pitta), but slow, methodical thinking (Kapha). Emotional: Passionate and nurturing; anger and attachment may arise when imbalanced. Kapha-Vata Characteristics Physical:

Ayurvedic yoga lifestyle for winter

Broad build (Kapha) but prone to coldness and dryness (Vata). Mental: Thoughtful and imaginative but inconsistent in focus.
Emotional: Calm and nurturing (Kapha), with occasional anxiety (Vata).

5. Sama Dosha (Balanced State)

Definition: When Vata, Pitta, and Kapha are in perfect harmony, the individual exhibits a balanced constitution.
Physical Characteristics: Healthy weight, glowing skin, excellent digestion.
Mental: Calm, sharp, and consistent thoughts.
Emotional: Even-tempered, compassionate, and confident.
Energy: Sustained and steady throughout the day.
Rare: True Sama Dosha is rare and requires careful lifestyle practices.

Ayurvedic yoga lifestyle for winter

AYURVEDIC RECIPES FOR WINTER

In Ayurveda, winter is characterised by cold, heavy, and damp qualities, making it a Kapha-dominant season. These seasonal attributes can aggravate both Vata and Kapha doshas. Winter is a time when nature slows down, reflecting the Kapha qualities of stability, structure, and endurance. However, the impact of winter varies across the three doshas—Vata, Pitta, and Kapha—depending on their inherent qualities and tendencies.

Kapha in Winter

Winter's cold and wet environment amplifies Kapha dosha, which is naturally composed of the earth (Prithvi) and water (Jala) elements. When balanced, Kapha provides strength, stability, and immunity during this season. However, if aggravated, it can lead to sluggishness, congestion, weight gain, and other Kapha-related imbalances. To maintain equilibrium, it is essential to embrace light, warmth, and invigorating practices. Spicy, bitter, and astringent foods, as well as activities that generate heat and movement, help balance Kapha during winter.

Ayurvedic yoga lifestyle for winter

Vata in Winter

Vata dosha, made up of air (Vayu) and ether (Akasha) elements, is inherently cold, dry, and light. While winter's moisture may temporarily calm Vata, its cold and dry qualities can aggravate this dosha if not appropriately managed. This can lead to issues like dry skin, joint stiffness, and increased anxiety. To counterbalance these effects, Vata individuals should focus on warmth, hydration, and grounding practices. Consuming warm, oily, and nourishing foods like soups, stews, and spiced teas is particularly beneficial. Nourishing foods like soups, stews, and spiced teas are particularly beneficial.

Pitta in Winter

Pitta dosha, governed by fire (Agni) and water (Jala) elements, generally remains stable during winter. The season's coolness naturally tempers Pitta's heat and intensity,
offering a period of balance. However, if Pitta is already aggravated, individuals may still experience symptoms like irritation or digestive issues. To support balance, Pitta individuals should continue to emphasize cooling yet nourishing foods, such as mildly spiced, sweet, and bitter options, while avoiding excessively hot or oily meals.

Ayurvedic yoga lifestyle for winter

In Ayurveda, the best time to eat sweets or dessert in winter is typically mid-morning or early afternoon, ideally after the digestive fire (Agni) has been well-kindled but not overloaded. The body's natural effort to maintain warmth causes the digestive fire to be more substantial during winter. This is the perfect time to indulge in more indulgent and heavier foods, including sweets.

Mid-morning (10 a.m. to 11:30 a.m.) is the ideal time for sweets. The Agni is active but not at its peak. This allows for proper digestion without overwhelming the system.
Early Afternoon (12 p.m. to 2 p.m.): After lunch or as part of the meal, the body can handle heavier or richer foods.
Avoid Eating Sweets at Night advises against consuming sweets late in the evening or at night, as digestion slows down. Eating sweets before bed can lead to ama (toxins) building up and sluggishness. If you are craving sweets, then Pairing Matters.
To balance the Kapha and Vata doshas dominant in winter, prefer warming, spiced desserts (e.g., with cinnamon, cardamom, or ginger). Avoid cold, heavy desserts like ice cream with warming spices unless consumed during the day.

Ayurvedic yoga lifestyle for winter

Breakfast
Warm Apple Cinnamon Porridge

Ingredients

Oats – 1/2 cup

Almond milk or water – 1 cup

Apples – 1 small (diced)

Cinnamon powder – 1/2 tsp

Cardamom powder – a pinch

Ghee – 1 tsp

Jaggery – to taste

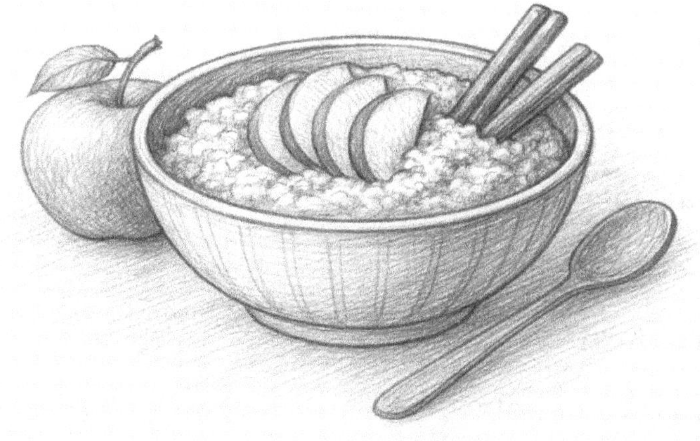

Ayurvedic yoga lifestyle for winter

Preparation

Cook oats with almond milk or water until soft.
In a pan, sauté dice apples in ghee and add
cinnamon and cardamom.
Mix the apples into the porridge and sweeten
with jaggery or honey.
Properties and Dosha Advantage:
Vata and Kapha pacifying: Warm, sweet, and
lightly spiced.
Pitta neutral: Non-heating spices balance
digestion.
Gunas: Light (Laghu), moist (Snigdha), and
grounding

Mid-Morning Snack

Roasted Sweet Potatoes with Cumin

Ingredients

Sweet potatoes – 1 cup (cubed)

Ghee or olive oil – 1 tsp

Cumin powder – 1/2 tsp

Black pepper – a pinch

Rock salt – to taste

Preparation:

Toss sweet potato cubes with ghee, cumin,
black pepper, and salt.

Ayurvedic yoga lifestyle for winter

Roast in the oven at 375°F (190°C) until soft and golden.

Mid-Morning Snack

ROASTED SWEET POTATOES WITH CUMIN

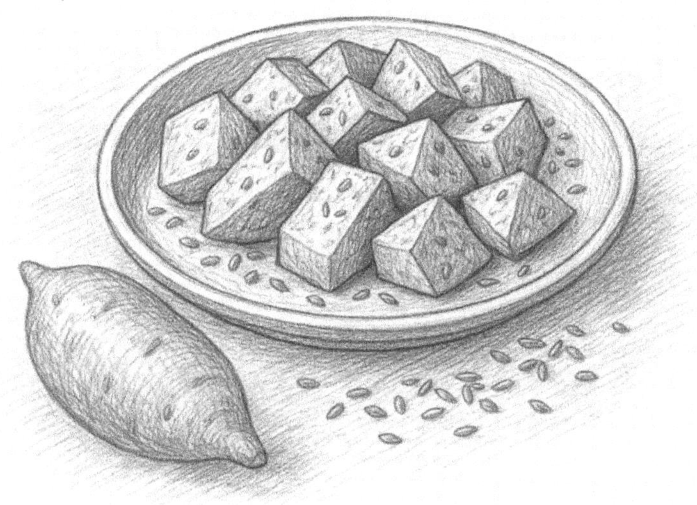

Properties and Dosha Advantage:
Vata pacifying: Sweet potatoes are grounding and moist.
Kapha balancing: Spices like cumin and pepper prevent heaviness.
Gunas: Nourishing (Snigdha), warm (Ushna).

Ayurvedic yoga lifestyle for winter

Lunch
Lentil Soup with Seasonal Vegetables

Ingredients:

Yellow moong dal – 1/2 cup (soaked)

Seasonal vegetables (carrots, zucchini, spinach) – 1 cup

Ghee – 1 tbsp

Cumin seeds – 1/2 tsp

Turmeric – 1/4 tsp

Ginger – 1/2 tsp (grated)

Rock salt – to taste

Preparation

Cook moong dal with vegetables until soft like soup
Heat ghee, sauté cumin seeds, turmeric, and ginger in a pan. Then temper the spices into the soup and stir well.

Ayurvedic yoga lifestyle for winter

Lentil Soup with Seasonal Vegetables

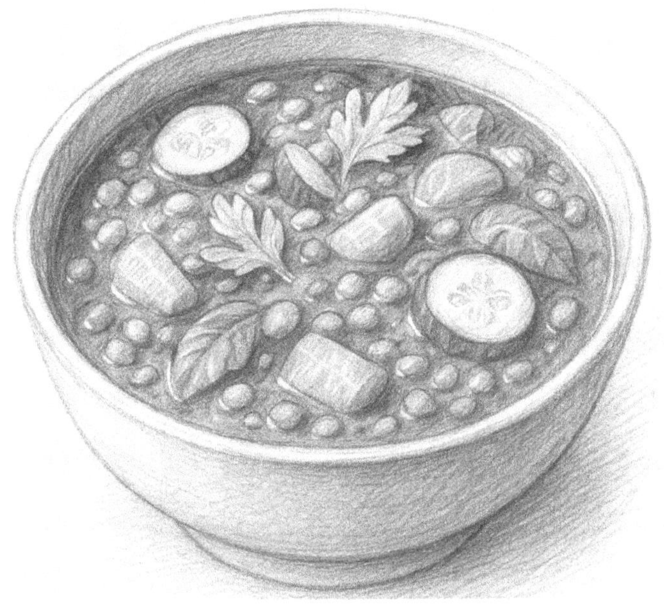

Properties and Dosha Advantage:
Vata and Kapha balancing: Warm, light, and easy to digest.
Pitta neutral: Gentle spices support Agni (digestive fire).
Gunas: Light (Laghu), warm (Ushna), and moist (Snigdha).

Ayurvedic yoga lifestyle for winter

Afternoon Drink
Spiced Golden Milk

Gold milk, also known as turmeric milk (Haldi Doodh), is a powerful Ayurvedic drink made by combining milk with turmeric and other warming spices like black pepper, cinnamon, and ginger. It has been used for centuries in Ayurveda for its numerous health benefits.

Ingredients

Milk (or almond milk) – 1 cup

Turmeric – 1/4 tsp

Ginger powder – a pinch

Black pepper – a pinch

Ghee – 1 tsp

Jaggery – to taste

Preparation

Heat milk with turmeric, ginger powder, and black pepper.
Add ghee and sweeten with jaggery

Ayurvedic Properties

Rasa (Taste): Bitter, Astringent, Pungent
Virya (Potency): Ushna (Hot)
Vipaka (Post-digestive Effect): Katu (Pungent)

Ayurvedic yoga lifestyle for winter

Guna (Qualities): Laghu (Light), Ruksha (Dry), Tikshna (Sharp Dosha)

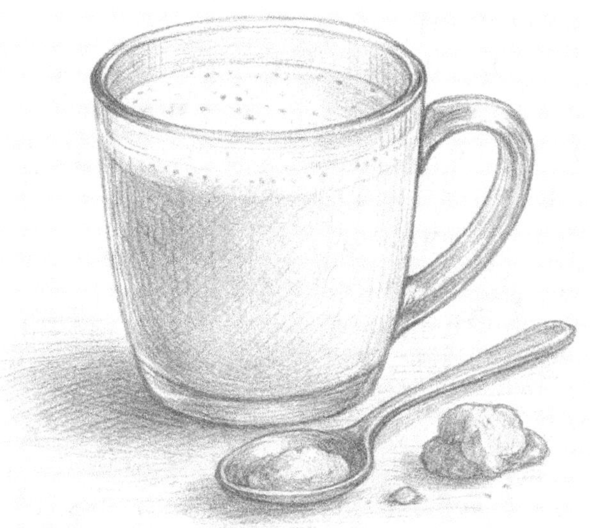

Afternoon Drink
Spiced Golden Milk

For Pitta Dosha

Advantages of Gold Milk

For Vata Dosha
It helps with joint pain, arthritis, and nerve-related issues. Improves digestion and reduces bloating. Provides warmth and stability for the mind and body.
If taken in moderation, it can aid in liver detoxification. Excessive consumption may

Ayurvedic yoga lifestyle for winter

aggravate Pitta due to turmeric's heating nature. Improves digestion and reduces bloating. Provides warmth and stability for the mind and body.

For Pitta Dosha, if taken in moderation, turmeric can aid in liver detoxification.

Excessive Consumption may aggravate Pitta due to its heating nature.

Best consumed with cooling herbs like fennel or cardamom to balance Pitta.

For Kapha Dosha

Help with clearing mucus and congestion. Supports weight management by improving metabolism. Acts as an immunity booster and prevents seasonal illnesses.

Dinner
Sweet Potato and Carrot Soup

Ingredients

Sweet potatoes – 1 cup (peeled and diced)

Carrots – 1 cup (peeled and diced)

Coconut milk – 1/2 cup

Ghee – 1 tbsp

Ginger – 1/2 tsp (grated)

Cumin powder – 1/2 tsp

Turmeric – 1/4 tsp

Ayurvedic yoga lifestyle for winter

Black pepper – a pinch

Rock salt – to taste

Water – 2 cups

Fresh coriander leaves – for garnish.

Preparation: Heat ghee in a pot and sauté grated ginger until aromatic. Add cumin powder, turmeric, and black pepper, and stir briefly to release their flavors. Next, add

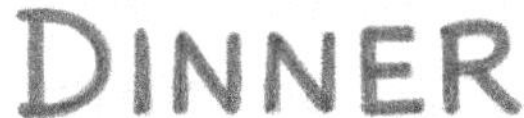

DINNER

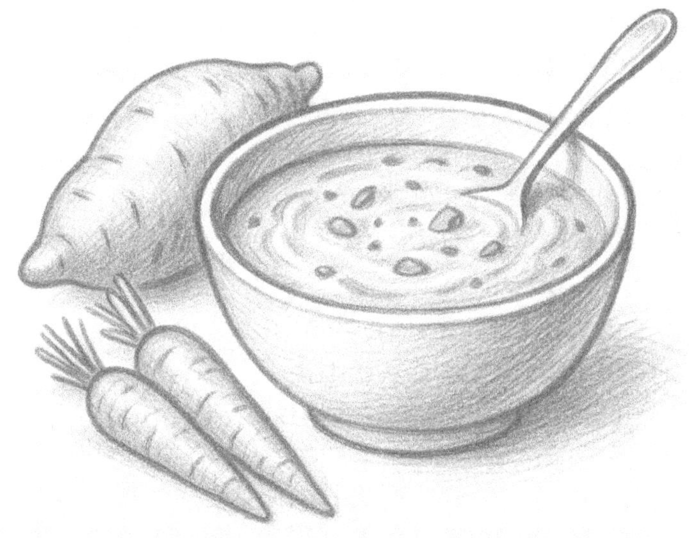

SWEET POTATO AND CARROT SOUP

Ayurvedic yoga lifestyle for winter

diced sweet potatoes and carrots, and sauté for 2–3 minutes. Pour in water, add rock salt, and then simmer until the vegetables are soft. Blend the soup until creamy using an immersion blender or in batches with a stand blender. Stir in coconut milk and allow it to simmer for 3–5 minutes. Finally, garnish with fresh coriander leaves before serving.

Properties and Dosha Advantage
Vata Pacifying: The warm soup provides grounding and hydration for the dry winter months.
Kapha Balancing: Light spices and warm cooking prevent heaviness and improve digestion.
Pitta Neutral: Gentle spices and the natural sweetness of carrots and sweet potatoes keep it soothing for Pitta.
Gunas: Warm (Ushna): Promotes internal warmth during cold weather.
Moist (Snigdha): Prevents dryness and supports hydration.
Light (Laghu): Easily digestible, ideal for an evening meal. This vibrant, nourishing soup is perfect for cold winter nights and supports all doshas.

The next item on the list is almond milk spiced with nutmeg and cardamom. It can be used to balance the doshas and promote good sleep. Warm Spiced Almond Milk with Nutmeg and Cardamom is an ideal Ayurvedic dish to encourage good sleep, balance the doshas, and ease digestion before bed. This dish soothes the nervous system, balances Vata and Pitta doshas, and mildly soothes Kapha dosha, making it perfect for restful sleep.

Warm Spiced Almond Milk

Ingredients

Organic almond milk -1 cup

(or cow's milk, if preferred and tolerated)

Nutmeg powder -1/4 tsp

(induces sleep and calms Vata)

Cardamom powder -1/4 tsp

(balances Kapha and adds warmth)

Cinnamon powder -1/4 tsp

(supports digestion)

Preparation

Gently heat the almond milk in a small pan over low heat, ensuring it does not boil. Add nutmeg, cardamom, cinnamon, and saffron (if using), and stir well. Allow the spices to

Ayurvedic yoga lifestyle for winter

steep for 2-3 minutes as the milk warms. Remove from heat, then add ghee (optional) and mix thoroughly. Let the milk cool slightly before adding honey (if using) to preserve its natural properties. Serve warm.

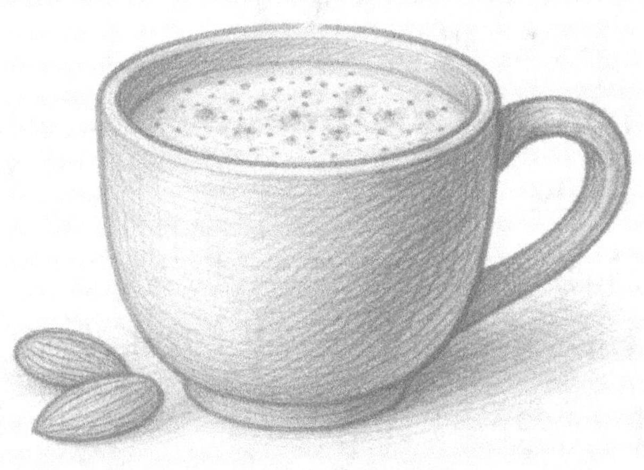

WARM SPICED ALMOND MILK

Why It Works for Sleep and Doshas
Vata Dosha: Warm milk and nutmeg soothe the nervous system, grounding the restlessness qualities of Vata.
Pitta Dosha: Cooling saffron and cardamom calm the mind and body, reducing excess heat or overthinking tendencies.
Kapha Dosha: The spices like cinnamon and cardamom add warmth and prevent

Ayurvedic yoga lifestyle for winter

heaviness, which can aggravate Kapha.

Additional Tips: Drink it about 30 minutes before bed. Ensure the environment is calm, dim, and free of stimulating activities to enhance the effect. Avoid consuming this if you feel overly full or if your digestion is sluggish. This Ayurvedic drink is light yet nourishing, helping you unwind and achieve deep, restorative sleep.

The winter season's final dish is a dessert that can be substituted for mid-morning snacks. It's a one-of-a-kind recipe for those who have a sweet tooth

Dessert Optional
Sesame Ladoo

Ingredients

White sesame seeds – 1/2 cup

Jaggery – 1/4 cup (grated)

Cardamom powder – a pinch

Ghee – 1 tsp

Preparation

Dry roast the sesame seeds until they turn golden and release a nutty aroma. In a pan,

Ayurvedic yoga lifestyle for winter

melt jaggery with ghee, stirring until smooth, then combine it with the roasted sesame seeds. Quickly shape the mixture into small balls while it is warm, and allow them to cool before serving

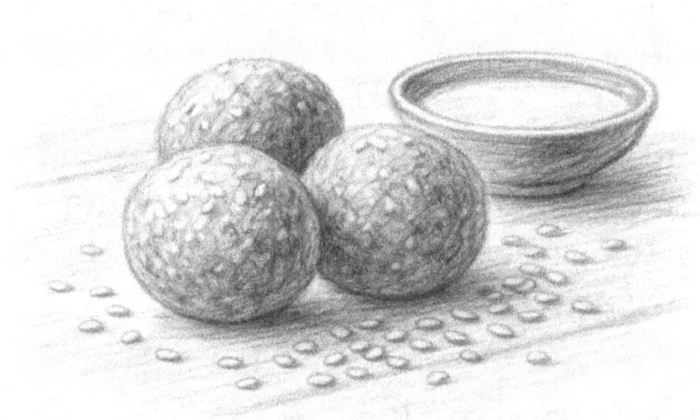

Dessert Optional
Sesame Ladoo

Properties and Dosha Advantage

Vata pacifying: Sesame seeds are grounding and nourishing. Kapha balancing: Warming
spices and ghee aid digestion.
Pitta neutral: Sweet and mildly spiced.
Gunas: Nourishing (Snigdha), grounding (Guru).

Ayurvedic yoga lifestyle for winter

1. Ginger-Tulsi Tea (for warming and immunity)

Benefits: Boosts immunity, supports digestion, and helps clear congestion.

Ingredients:

- 1-inch fresh ginger (sliced or grated)
- 1 tsp dried Tulsi (Holy Basil) or 4-5 fresh leaves
- One cup water
- Optional: a slice of lemon and honey (add after steeping)

How to prepare: Boil the ginger in water for 5 minutes, then add Tulsi and steep for another 3–5 minutes. Strain and enjoy.

2. Cinnamon-Cardamom-Clove Tea (warming and circulatory support)

Benefits: Warms the body, enhances circulation, and supports respiratory health.

Ingredients:

- 1 cinnamon stick
- 3 green cardamom pods
- 2 whole cloves

Ayurvedic yoga lifestyle for winter

- 1 cup water

How to prepare: Simmer all the spices in water for 10 minutes. Strain and sip warm. You can sweeten it with a little jaggery or honey if desired.

3. Licorice-Fennel Tea (soothing and balancing)

Benefits: Soothes dry throat, calms Vata, aids digestion, and supports respiratory health.

Ingredients:

- 1 tsp dried licorice root (Yashtimadhu)

- 1 tsp fennel seeds

- 1 cup water

How to prepare:
Simmer the licorice root and fennel seeds in water for 5–7 minutes. Strain and sip slowly. Avoid excessive use of licorice if you have high blood pressure.

4. Ashwagandha Rose Tea (nourishing and calming)

Benefits: Rejuvenates the nervous system, combats stress, and balances hormones—great for winter's mental fatigue and low energy.

Ayurvedic yoga lifestyle for winter

Ingredients:

- ½ tsp Ashwagandha powder

- 1 tsp dried rose petals or a rosebud tea

- 1 cup hot water

- Optional: a few drops of rose water or a splash of almond milk

- **How to prepare:**
  Steep rose petals in hot water for 5 minutes, then stir in Ashwagandha powder until dissolved. Strain (if needed) and enjoy.

Vegetables Best for Winter

VEGETABLES	BEST FOR	QUALITY
Sweet Potatoes	Vata, Pitta	Heavy, grounding, slightly sweet and warming
Carrots	Vata, Kapha	Sweet and slightly warm; good in soups/stews
Beets	Vata, Pitta	Builds blood, grounding, supports liver

Ayurvedic yoga lifestyle for winter

Pumpkin	Vata, Pitta	Nourishing, easy to digest, sweet
Spinach) (cooked)	Kapha, Pitta	Slightly bitter, lightens Kapha, avoid raw in winter
Cauliflower	Kapha	Light and astringent, balancing for Kapha, but cook well for Vata
Onions & Garlic	Vata, Kapha	Warming, improving circulation, detoxifying
Turnips & Rutabaga	Vata, Kapha	Earthy, grounding, especially good roasted

Fruits Best for Winter

FRUIT	BEST FOR	QUALITY
Apples (cooked)	Kapa, Pitta	Baked or stewed; grounding and gently detoxifying

Ayurvedic yoga lifestyle for winter

Pears (ripe/cooked)	Vata, Pitta	Soothing to digestion; moist and sweet
Dates & Figs	Vata	Nourishing, energy-boosting, excellent in warm drinks or porridges
Bananas (ripe)	Vata	Moistening and grounding, but avoid if Kapha is high
Pomegranates	Kapha, Pitta	Light and astringent; juice supports heart and liver
Oranges (sweet ones)	Kapha	Add zest and warmth, but avoid sour types for Vata
Avocados	Vata	Oily and grounding, good in moderation

Ayurvedic yoga lifestyle for winter

		for winter nourishment

Key Guidelines for Winter Meals

- **Favor Warm, Cooked Foods:** Avoid cold and raw foods to maintain digestive fire (Agni).
- **Use Warming Spices:** Include ginger, turmeric, cinnamon, cumin, and black pepper.
- **Nourish with Healthy Fats:** Ghee and sesame oil provide warmth and lubrication.
- **Balance Sweet and Spicy Tastes:** Sweet for grounding Vata and spicy for stimulating Kapha.

General Ayurvedic Tips for Winter Diet:

Focus on warm, cooked, and lightly spiced foods that are easy to digest. Minimize cold, raw, or overly heavy meals.

Lifestyle: Engage in regular physical activity to counteract Kapha's sluggish tendencies. Prioritise warmth and comfort to manage Vata.

Self-Care: Practice oil massages (Abhyanga) with warming oils like sesame or almond to keep the body hydrated and supple.

Routine: Maintain a consistent daily schedule, as regularity helps keep all doshas balanced

Ayurvedic yoga lifestyle for winter

during the winter months. By understanding how winter influences each dosha and adopting seasonally appropriate practices, individuals can maintain harmony and well-being throughout this Kapha-dominant season.

Ayurvedic yoga lifestyle for winter

COMMON WINTER CHALLENGES

Doshas in Winter

Winter's cold, dry, and windy characteristics make Vata Dosha more susceptible to imbalance. Managing Vata becomes crucial in early winter to maintain harmony and prevent discomfort.

As the winter season progresses, Kapha dosha slowly builds up due to the increasing cold and dampness in the environment. While Vata dominates the early winter months, Kapha subtly rises in the latter half, signaling the need for balancing strategies to adapt to this seasonal shift.

Strength and Qualities of the Body in Winter

The digestive fire (Agni) becomes more potent in winter because the external cold prevents body heat from dissipating outward, preserving warmth within the body. This internal heat improves digestion, allowing the body to process food more effectively.

The body can retain heat inside because cold weather can cause blockages in its external

Ayurvedic yoga lifestyle for winter

channels (such as sweat glands). While this can enhance digestion, Vata's inherent dryness and mobility can worsen if not balanced correctly.

Consuming sufficient food counters Vata's light and dry qualities. If the body does not get enough nourishment, Rasa Dhatu (the first product of digestion that nourishes all tissues) becomes depleted. This leads to Vata imbalance, causing symptoms such as bloating, gastritis, body aches, headaches, and joint pain.

This may explain why people naturally crave heavier, fatty foods like fondue, raclette, and Rösti during winter in Switzerland, as this helps pacify Vata dosha. People worldwide celebrate many festive occasions in the winter, such as Christmas, Ramadan, and Deevali. However, it is essential to ensure balanced nutrition to avoid excess Kapha accumulation later in the season. You can take control of your health and well-being by understanding and practicing this.

Impact of Winter on the Lymphatic System (Rasa Dhatu)

Kapha Influence

- Characteristics of Kapha: Cold, heavy, stable, and moist.
- Effects on the Lymphatic System:

Ayurvedic yoga lifestyle for winter

- Sluggish Movement: Kapha's heavy and stable nature can cause stagnation in the lymphatic flow, leading to fluid retention, swelling, and reduced detoxification efficiency.
- Mucus Accumulation: Kapha dominance can increase mucus production, which may result in blockages in lymphatic pathways and respiratory congestion.
- Weakened Agni (Digestive Fire): The slow metabolic processes associated with Kapha can reduce the body's ability to process waste, placing additional strain on the lymphatic system.

Vata Influence

- Characteristics: Cold, dry, light, and mobile.
- Effects on the Lymphatic System:
- Dryness in Tissues: Vata's dry quality can dehydrate the lymphatic fluid, leading to thicker lymph that circulates less efficiently.
- Increased Sensitivity: Vata dominance can exacerbate nervous system responses, creating an imbalance that affects the immune regulation managed by the lymphatic system.

Ayurvedic yoga lifestyle for winter

- Irregular Flow: Vata's mobile and erratic nature can disrupt the consistent movement of lymph, causing localized imbalances or blockages.

Reduced Circulation

Winter's cold temperatures can cause blood vessels to constrict, a process known as vasoconstriction. This constriction slows blood flow and lymphatic fluid, making it harder for the lymphatic system to efficiently remove toxins and waste from the body. Physical activity, which promotes lymph flow, is also often reduced in colder months, further contributing to sluggish lymphatic circulation.

This reduced circulation can be more pronounced in older individuals, as natural age-related declines in circulation compound the effects of cold weather. Weakened **Immunity**

The lymphatic system houses lymph nodes, which filter harmful pathogens and produce immune cells to fight infections. In winter, the body is more susceptible to colds, flu, and other respiratory infections due to increased time spent indoors and closer proximity to others. This heightened exposure to pathogens can overload the lymphatic system, particularly in older adults whose immune responses may already be compromised due to ageing.

Reduced Hydration

Lack of hydration can cause decreased thirst and water intake in cold weather, leading to mild dehydration. The lymphatic system relies on adequate hydration to maintain the fluidity of lymph. Lymphatic fluid can become thicker and harder to circulate if you don't drink enough water, slowing the detoxification process and affecting overall immunity.

Skin and Lymphatic Drainage

Winter often brings dry skin due to lower humidity and indoor heating, which can reduce the body's ability to eliminate toxins through sweating. Sweat glands are a secondary means of detoxification, and when they are less active, the lymphatic system must compensate. This effect can strain the lymphatic system of older adults, whose skin naturally becomes drier and thinner with age.

Why Age Matters

The lymphatic system's efficiency naturally declines as we age due to reduced muscle tone, lower metabolic rates, and decreased overall immune function. Winter intensifies these challenges, making it harder for older individuals to maintain optimal lymphatic health. Reduced circulation, dehydration, and a

Ayurvedic yoga lifestyle for winter

less active lifestyle in colder months compound the strain on an ageing lymphatic system, making it less effective at fighting infections and removing toxins.

Ayurvedic yoga lifestyle for winter

SEASONAL WELLNESS GUIDE

Ritucharya for Winter (Hemanta and Shishira)

Ritucharya, the Ayurvedic seasonal regimen, is so important in Ayurveda. It provides guidelines for aligning your lifestyle, diet, and habits with seasonal changes to maintain optimal health.

Winter is divided into two sub-seasons: Hemanta (early winter) and Shishira (late winter). During these periods, the body's digestive fire (Agni) is at its strongest, making it ideal for nourishing the body and building strength.

Hemanta Ritucharya (Early Winter)

This phase is often marked by moderate cold and dry weather from mid-November to mid-January. Aligning routines with the season, weather, and geography is crucial for maintaining health. However, seasonal patterns may vary. For example, November may experience peak winter due to climate change. Your overall well-being is dependent on adapting your lifestyle to these changing conditions.

Ayurvedic yoga lifestyle for winter

Seasons can vary depending on the hemisphere you live in, so adjusting your seasonal routine to maintain balance and well-being is essential.

People typically follow lifestyles shaped by what they learned in childhood or what makes them feel relaxed. In the past, humans preferred to live in environments with the weather and geography they were accustomed to when they moved or travelled. They adapted their lifestyle to the new conditions; failing to do so often led to health problems or even death. This highlights the importance of aligning one's lifestyle with the seasons and local climate.

Nowadays, people are exploring different cultures, weather and geographies, and learning how to adjust and maintain one's life is crucial. Flexibility is key—without it, you risk losing your physical and mental fitness, making life more challenging.

Ayurvedic yoga lifestyle for winter

RITUCHARYA FOR WINTER SYNCHRONIZING

Adapting ensures you can fully enjoy and explore the beauty of life with joy and vitality.

Ritucharya

Make nutrition a priority, including warming spices, eating healthy fats, consuming warm foods, staying away from cold, and adjusting your overall lifestyle for winter. Include seasonal produce like root vegetables. The use of warming spices can enhance the immune system and digestion.

Lifestyle Corrections

Daily Oil Massage (Abhyanga): Use warm oils like sesame oil to protect the skin from dryness and improve circulation.

Physical Activity: Engage in exercise or yoga to maintain flexibility and warmth.

Clothing: Wear warm, insulated clothes to shield yourself from the cold air.

One valuable lesson we can learn from the Swiss is how they encourage their children to experience all types of weather, including extreme conditions. They believe that the

Ayurvedic yoga lifestyle for winter

weather is just a part of life, and with proper clothing, the body can be protected while fully

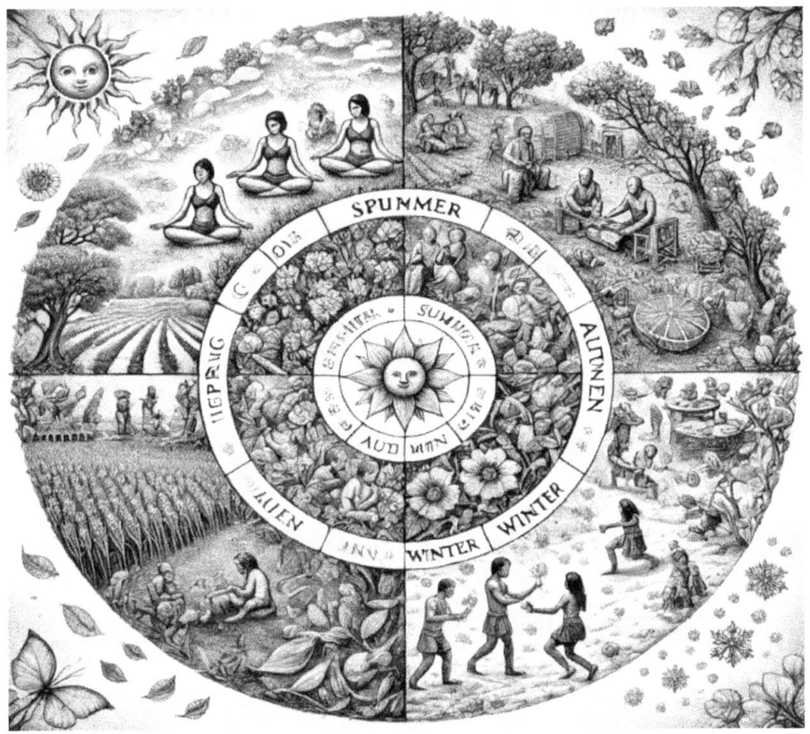

enjoying the outdoors. This mindset is complemented by engaging in winter activities tailored to the season.

Similarly, Scandinavian countries follow a fascinating practice: they let toddlers nap in strollers (kinderwagens) outdoors, even during winter. Surprisingly, the children sleep comfortably because they are dressed appropriately. This practice is believed to strengthen their immunity against the cold.

Ayurvedic yoga lifestyle for winter

The key takeaway is to embrace fitness and seasonal activities suitable for the weather, allowing you to enjoy and adapt to each season. For more insights on integrating such practices into your lifestyle, refer to the chapter on Dinacharya (daily routines).

Shishira Ritucharya (Late Winter)

This phase usually spans from mid-January to mid-March and is characterized by extreme cold and dampness

Strengthen Immunity: Continue eating warm, nutritious meals, but focus more on boosting immunity. add herbs like ashwagandha, Tulsi, and Mulethi (liquorice root) to your diet.

Combat Kapha Accumulation:

As Kapha dosha starts increasing, reduce excessively oily or heavy foods. opt for lighter meals like soups and stews.

Limit Sweet and Cold Foods: Reduce sugar and dairy intake to prevent Kapha imbalance.

Lifestyle - According to Dinachariya

Strengthen, maintain mental balance, and prepare your body to thrive throughout the season. (Explain to the next chapter.) Following a structured daily routine to soothe Vata's

Ayurvedic yoga lifestyle for winter

uncontrollable nature and stabilize Kapha (Dinacharya). Get enough sleep to enable the lymphatic system to regenerate and function optimally.

Ayurvedic yoga lifestyle for winter

INNER CLOCK WITH DINACHARYA

Dinacharya

Our body operates on a natural rhythm called the circadian clock, which governs various biological processes. Ayurveda emphasizes the importance of aligning this inner clock with nature's cycles through Dinacharya daily routine designed to harmonize our body, mind, and environment. Synchronizing your inner clock with Dinacharya is especially crucial during seasonal transitions, such as winter, when external changes can disrupt balance.

Why is synchronising the Inner Clock Important?

Supports Natural Rhythms:

Dinacharya helps align our body with the Earth's cycles, ensuring smoother transitions through day and night. This alignment improves digestion, sleep, and energy levels.

Boosts Immunity:

A structured daily routine strengthens the immune system, protecting the body from seasonal illnesses such as colds and respiratory infections.

Enhances Mental Clarity:

Ayurvedic yoga lifestyle for winter

Consistency in daily habits reduces stress, improves focus, and promotes emotional well-being.

Balances Doshas

Dinacharya ensures that doshas like Vata, Pitta, and Kapha remain in equilibrium, preventing seasonal imbalances that can lead to health issues.

Key Elements of Dinacharya for Synchronising the Inner Clock

Wake Up with Nature:

Rise early, ideally before sunrise (around 5:30–6:00 a.m.), to synchronize with the Vata phase of the day, which supports alertness and energy.

Morning Detox:

Start your day with cleansing practices such as:

Tongue scraping to remove toxins (ama). Drinking warm water with lemon or herbal tea stimulates digestion.

Daily Oil Massage (Abhyanga):

In the morning, perform a warm oil massage to ground the body and calm the nervous system.

Physical Activity:

Ayurvedic yoga lifestyle for winter

Engage in light exercise or yoga to activate your metabolism and maintain flexibility, especially in colder months.

Eat According to the Clock:

Follow a routine of regular, balanced meals:
A substantial breakfast (7-8 a.m.) to fuel the day.
A hearty lunch (12-1 p.m.) when digestion is strongest.
A lighter dinner (6–7 p.m.) to prepare for restful sleep.
Respect the Evening Wind-Down:
As the day transitions into night, it reduces mental and physical activity to prepare for sleep.
Avoid stimulating activities like screen time after 8 p.m.
Sleeping with the Natural Cycle:
Go to bed early (ideally by 10 p.m.) for 7–8 hours of restorative sleep. This aligns with the Kapha phase of the night, promoting deep rest.

Benefits of a Well-Synchronised Inner Clock

- Improved digestion and metabolism.
- Enhanced immunity and resilience to seasonal ailments.
- Better energy levels and focus throughout the day.

Ayurvedic yoga lifestyle for winter

- Reduced stress and improved emotional stability.
- Balanced doshas lead to overall wellness.

Following Dinacharya, you honour your body's inner clock, creating a foundation for health and harmony, especially during the demanding winter.

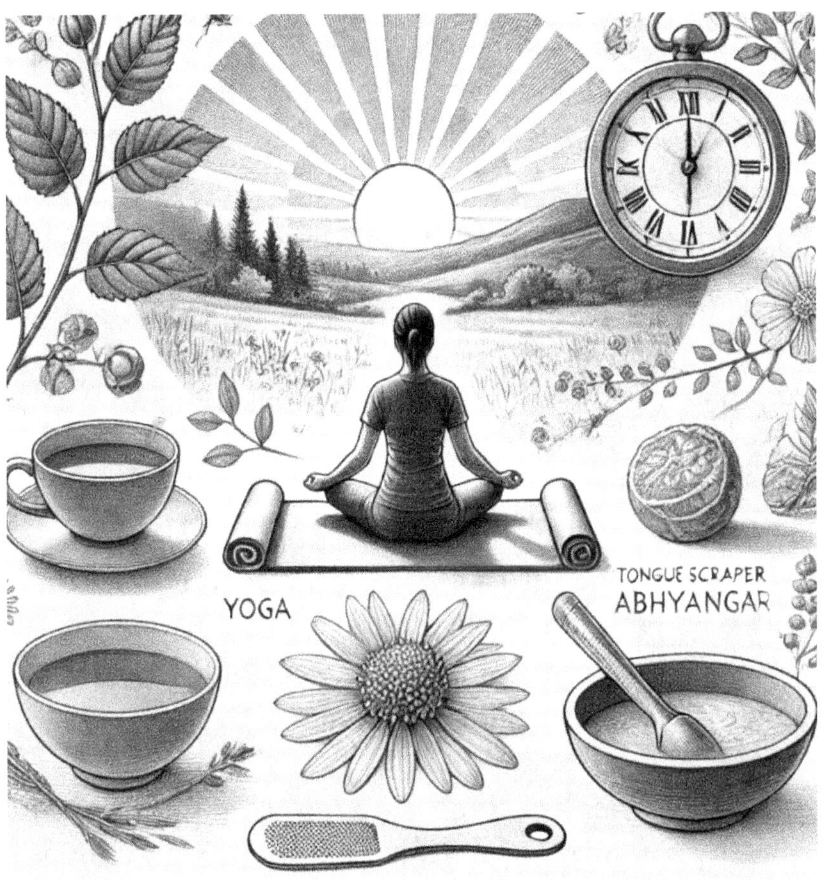

Ayurvedic yoga lifestyle for winter

WINTER MEDITATION

Winter is a season often associated with introspection, rest, and finding balance as nature slows down and enters a quieter phase. Winter meditation, focusing on stillness and reflection, can help bring balance by allowing you to attune to your body, mind, and emotions in a way that nurtures grounding, peace, and restoration. Here are a few specific winter meditations, with explanations, that can bring balance:

The Grounding Meditation: "Root to Earth"

Winter can feel like a time of withdrawal, and grounding meditations help us feel connected to the earth beneath us, even in the cold and stillness of the season.

How to Practice:

- Settle into a comfortable seated position or lie down in a quiet, peaceful space."
- Close your eyes and take deep, slow breaths, allowing yourself to relax into the present moment.
- Visualise roots growing from the soles of your feet (or your tailbone if lying down) deep into the earth, extending through

Ayurvedic yoga lifestyle for winter

layers of soil and rock and into the centre of the earth.

- Feel the stability of the earth supporting you, like a steady foundation.
- With each breath, imagine drawing energy from the earth into your body, filling you with warmth, vitality, and balance.
- As you breathe out, release any tension or negative energy back into the earth, trusting it will be transformed.
- Keep practicing for 5 to 15 minutes. Initially, practice for 5 minutes and gradually increase your timing.

Benefits: This meditation promotes stability and connection to nature, often needed in the colder months when the natural world feels more dormant. It helps anchor your energy and provides a sense of security and calm during a season that can often feel isolated or heavy.

The Light Within Meditation: "Embrace the Inner Light"

Winter days are shorter, and the darkness can sometimes lead to feelings of fatigue or sadness. This meditation helps you connect with your inner light, a powerful source of warmth and positivity.

Ayurvedic yoga lifestyle for winter

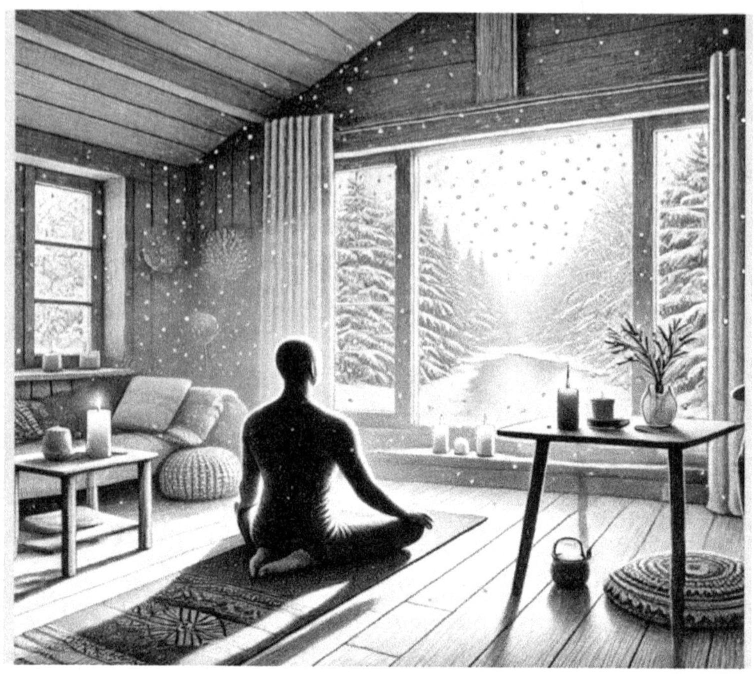

Winter Meditation

How to Practice:

- Sit comfortably, with your spine straight and hands resting on your lap.
- Breathe deeply a few times, letting your body relax more with each breath out.

Close your eyes and imagine a small, glowing light within your heart. It may be warm and golden or a cool, calming blue, whatever resonates with you.

- Close your eyes and imagine a small, glowing light within your heart. It may be

Ayurvedic yoga lifestyle for winter

warm and golden or a cool, calming blue, whatever resonates with you.

- As you inhale, imagine this light growing brighter and warmer, filling your chest with peaceful energy.
- With each exhale, feel any tension or negativity dissolve into the light, allowing the warmth to spread throughout your body.
- Visualize the light growing bigger, enveloping you in a protective aura of warmth and filling you with peace and steady energy through the cold season.
- Keep practicing for 5 to 15 minutes. Initially, practice for 5 minutes and gradually increase your timing

Benefits: This meditation reminds you that even during the darkest days of winter, there is always an inner light of warmth and vitality. It helps lift your mood, promotes self-compassion, and restores your energy.

Ayurvedic yoga lifestyle for winter

MENTAL HEALTH CHALLENGES

Winter can bring specific mental health challenges due to the changes in weather, daylight, and routine. For many, the colder months can feel isolating or difficult, and seasonal changes can trigger mental health issues such as Seasonal Affective Disorder (SAD), anxiety, and depression.

Seasonal Affective Disorder (SAD)

SAD is a type of depression that occurs at the same time every year, usually in the winter months. It is associated with a lack of sunlight and shorter days, which can affect mood-regulating chemicals in the brain, such as serotonin.

How Meditation Helps:

- Reduces Stress and Anxiety: Meditation can help lower cortisol levels, the stress hormone. Lower stress levels can alleviate some of the feelings of overwhelm that people with SAD might experience.
- Enhances Serotonin and Dopamine Production: Mindfulness practices, mainly

Ayurvedic yoga lifestyle for winter

focusing on positive thoughts or gratitude, can increase the production of feel-good neurotransmitters like serotonin and dopamine. These neurotransmitters play an important role in regulating mood and can combat depressive feelings.

- Promote Relaxation: Meditation can help calm the body's stress response, aiding in relaxation and improving sleep, which can be disrupted during winter

Meditation, Pranayama, consuming seasonal foods, and adhering to Ritucharya and Dinacharya practices can help maintain physical and mental well-being. These habits enable individuals to face seasonal changes and challenges with resilience, staying calm and joyful. Meditation empowers you to master your mind, fostering clarity and inner peace.

No one is immune to mental health challenges, and taking care of our mental well-being is a fundamental responsibility crucial to prioritising mental health during winter. Engage in activities that keep you active and uplift your mood, promoting a joyful state of mind. These practices also help maintain hormonal balance, contributing to overall happiness.

Ayurvedic yoga lifestyle for winter

By following a seasonal routine, staying flexible, and embracing activities that bring joy, you can make the most of winter while keeping your mind and body in harmony. Enjoy the season and nurture your happiness!

Vitamin D Deficiency

Shorter daylight hours and colder weather often limit outdoor activity during winter, decreasing Vitamin D production. This deficiency can contribute to feelings of fatigue, depression, and overall mental fatigue.

How Meditation Helps: Mindfulness to Enhance Self-Care: Meditation encourages you to check in with your body and mind, prompting you to take better care of yourself. Practising mindfulness can help you

- Pay attention to your energy levels, identify when you feel drained, and decide to recharge.
- Deep Breathing can help to energise the body and mind, helping mitigate the sluggishness that can result from Vitamin D deficiency.

Ayurvedic yoga lifestyle for winter

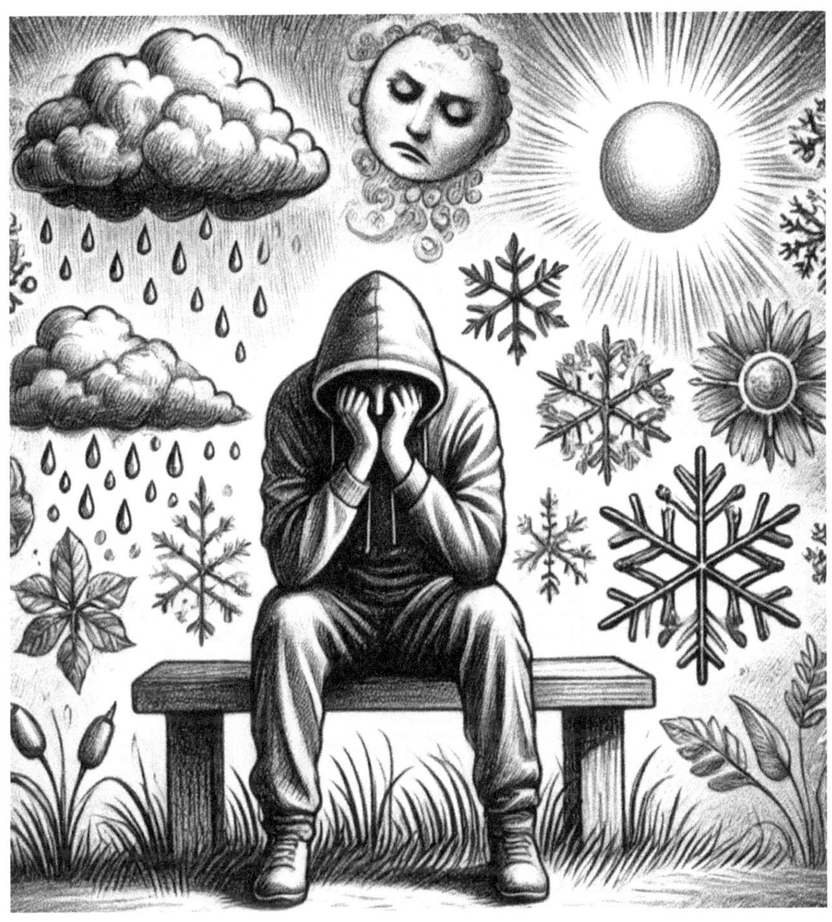

Sleep Issues

Shorter days and a lack of sunlight can disrupt sleep patterns, especially in winter. People with seasonal affective disorder may experience more severe sleep disturbances, including oversleeping or insomnia.

Ayurvedic yoga lifestyle for winter

How Meditation Helps

- Promote Better Sleep: Meditation helps calm the nervous system and reduce anxiety, making it easier to fall asleep. Guided meditation for sleep can encourage relaxation by relaxing the mind and releasing physical tension.
- Improve Sleep Quality: Deep relaxation and mindfulness before bedtime can promote more restful and restorative sleep. Practices such as progressive muscle relaxation and body scans can prepare the body for deep rest, which is essential for mental health

Ayurvedic yoga lifestyle for winter

WINTER PRANAYAM

Pranayama, which refers to the control of breath, is a central practice in yoga that can be especially beneficial during the winter months. Winter brings unique challenges for our physical and mental health, including the cold, low energy levels, dry air, and increased susceptibility to illness. Pranayama can help balance and regulate the body's internal systems, making it a valuable tool for maintaining health, energy, and emotional well-being in the winter.

Specific Pranayama Practices for Winter:

"I would like to explain three specific pranayama techniques that are especially beneficial during the winter months."

1. Bhastrika Pranayama (Bellows Breath)

Bhastrika is an energizing breath that stimulates the body's internal heat, increases circulation, and clears the airways. It's great for combating the cold and boosting energy during the winter months.

How to Practice Bhastrika:

- Sit comfortably in a cross-legged position or on a chair with your spine straight.
- Take a few slow, deep breaths, and feel your body loosen with every exhale.,
- Making the exhale active.
- Continue with short, powerful exhales and inhales, emphasising both equally.
  Start slowly, with 10 rounds, and gradually increase to 30-40 rounds

Ayurvedic yoga lifestyle for winter

- Focus on the breath and feel the warmth building in your body.

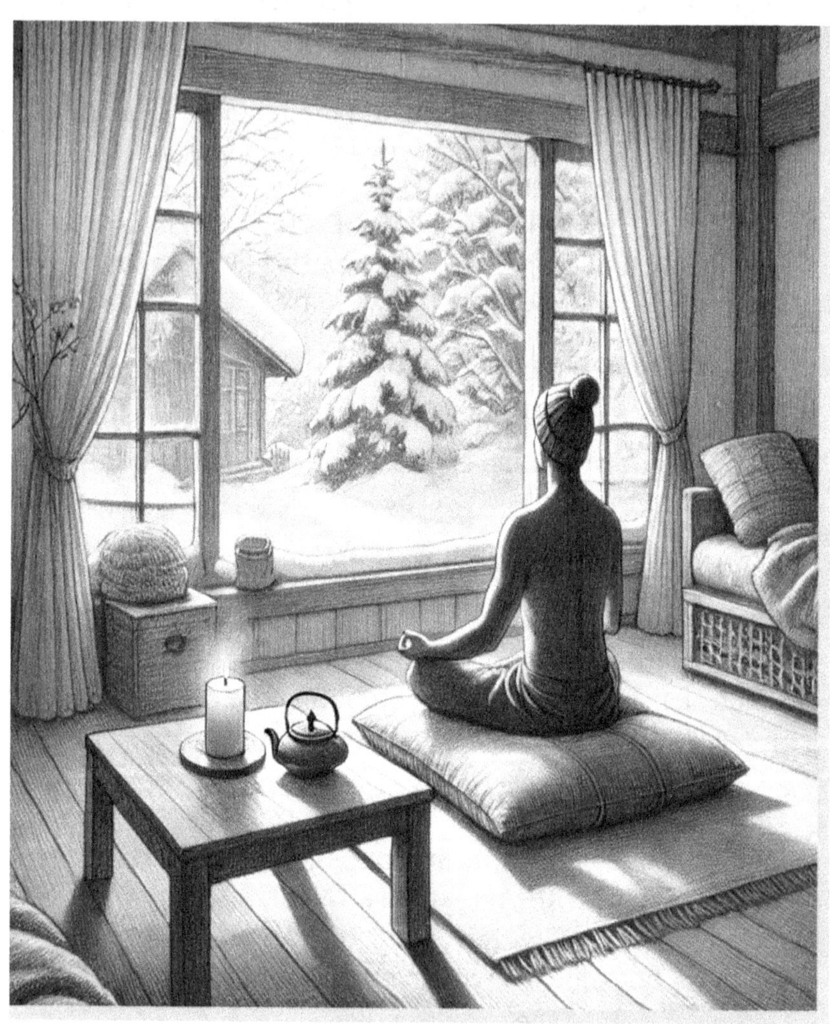

Ayurvedic yoga lifestyle for winter

Benefits for Winter:

- Warms the Body: The rapid breathing in Bhastrika generates heat, which helps combat the cold weather.
- Boosts Circulation: It increases blood flow to the brain and body, promoting warmth and energy.
- Clears the Respiratory Tract: It helps clear mucus or blockages in the respiratory system, making it helpful for those prone to respiratory issues in winter.

2. Kapalbhati Pranayama (Skull Shining Breath)

Kapalbhati is a cleansing breath that detoxifies the body and stimulates the digestive system. This pranayama also generates heat and is an excellent practice for boosting energy during the winter.

How to Practice Kapalbhati:

- Sit in a comfortable position with your spine straight and shoulders relaxed.
- Take a deep breath through your nose, then forcefully exhale through the nose,
- Engaging your abdominal muscles to push the air out.
- Let the breath come in naturally and gently push the air out with intention.
- Do these 20 to 30 times, then pause and simply notice your breathing.
- Keep your attention on your breathing and notice the heat rising within you.

Ayurvedic yoga lifestyle for winter

Benefits for Winter:

- **Generates Internal Heat**: Kapalbhati creates a warming sensation in the body, helping you stay warm in cold weather.
- **Clears the Sinuses**: It helps to clear blocked nasal passages, improving breathing and reducing the chances of colds and sinus congestion during the winter.
- **Stimulates Metabolism**: Rapid exhalations stimulate the digestive system, which can be sluggish in winter.

3.Anulom Vilom Pranayama (Nadi Shodhana or Alternate Nostril Breathing)

Anulom Vilom is a calming and balancing pranayama that promotes overall health, reduces stress, and improves mental clarity. It also effectively calms the nervous system, which can become overstimulated in the cold and dark winter months.

How to Practice Anulom Vilom:

- Sit in a comfortable, upright position.
- With ease, bring your thumb to your right nostril, softly closing it. Draw a deep, calming breath through your left nostril."
- Now, close your left nostril using your ring finger, release the right nostril, and breathe out slowly.
- Inhale through the right nostril, close it with your thumb, and exhale gently through the left nostril.

Ayurvedic yoga lifestyle for winter

- Continue this alternate nostril breathing for 5-10 minutes.

Benefits for Winter:

- Balances the Nervous System: This pranayama is soothing and grounding, helping to alleviate anxiety or stress that may be heightened during winter.
- Improves Oxygen Flow: Anulom Vilom clears blockages in the nasal passages, ensuring fresh, oxygenated air reaches the lungs, which can feel especially refreshing in winter.
- Reduces Dryness: Improving airflow through both nostrils can help humidify the respiratory system, alleviating dryness caused by the cold air. In winter, Pranayama practices can be a powerful way to address the physical and mental challenges that arise during the colder months. Specific pranayama techniques like Bhastrika, Kapalbhati, and Anulom Vilom have a good effect, generating internal warmth, improving circulation, enhancing immunity, and reducing stress. These practices help balance the body and mind, supporting overall well-being and energy levels when naturally feeling tired, cold, and withdrawn

If you want to know about many other pranayamas, please check our eBook, which is specifically for pranayama and meditation and provides more details.

Ayurvedic yoga lifestyle for winter

YOGA FOR WINTER

Why Yoga for Winter?

Yoga is traditionally practiced in alignment with the weather, temperature, and the practitioner's health and fitness conditions. The season and time of practice also play a crucial role in ensuring that practice benefits rather than harms the body. Different asanas (Yoga Poses) can be chosen based on the season, catering to the body's needs.

However, many modern yoga teachers are unaware of this nuanced approach. For example, if a Pitta-dominant person practices Surya Namaskar in the middle of the day during summer, it can aggravate their Pitta imbalance, potentially leading to digestive issues. Similarly, a senior individual with a Vata constitution who practices excessive standing asanas may exacerbate conditions like arthritis.

To protect and enhance your health, it is crucial to understand the timing, seasonal adjustments, and suitability of any fitness program, including yoga. If you face challenges with specific asanas, please check out our e-book, specifically on yoga poses, which will guide the basic level to advanced practitioners. but here in this book, I am going to explain ten yoga poses which are

Ayurvedic yoga lifestyle for winter

exclusively for winter; let us see why yoga poses are good for winter

Why yoga is ideal for winter

Improves Circulation and Warmth

- Cold Weather Effects: Cold weather can cause blood vessels to constrict, reducing circulation and leaving you feeling cold and stiff, especially in the hands, feet, and joints.
- Yoga Advantage: Yoga postures, particularly those that engage large muscle groups (like standing poses, backbends, and core strengthening asanas), increase circulation throughout the body. These movements promote the flow of oxygen-rich blood, helping to warm up the body from the inside out and reduce coldness, stiffness, or numbness in the extremities.

2. Boosts Immunity and Prevents Illness

- Cold and Flu Season: Winter is known for increasing illnesses, such as colds, flu, and respiratory infections. The immune system can be weakened during the winter due to changes in temperature, reduced sunlight, and lifestyle habits.

Ayurvedic yoga lifestyle for winter

- Yoga Advantage: Yoga can help strengthen the immune system. Specific postures, like chest openers and inversions, increase lymphatic flow and detoxification, promoting immune function. Breathing exercises (pranayama) improve lung capacity and help clear nasal passages, which are essential during winter's dry, cold air.

3. Increases Flexibility and Reduces Stiffness

Cold Weather Effects: Cold weather causes muscles and joints to become tighter and more prone to injury. Lack of movement during colder months can result in a loss of flexibility, leading to aches, stiffness, and even back pain.

- Yoga Advantage: Yoga helps counteract this stiffness by promoting flexibility through gentle stretches and dynamic movements. Poses like forward bends, twists, and hip openers improve joint mobility and muscle flexibility. The practice of yoga also increases blood flow to the muscles, helping to keep them limber and reducing tightness

4. Energy balance and Fights Winter Fatigue

- Winter Fatigue: The lack of sunlight reduces physical activity, and colder

Ayurvedic yoga lifestyle for winter

temperatures can lead to feelings of sluggishness and fatigue, making it harder to stay active and motivated during the winter months.

- Yoga Advantage: Yoga helps to boost energy and combat fatigue. Certain poses, such as backbends (like Cobra or Bow Pose) and standing poses (like Warrior I or Warrior II), activate the body and promote a sense of vitality. Pranayama practices, especially those focused on energizing breaths like Bhastrika (Bellows Breath) or Kapalbhati (Skull Shining Breath), increase alertness and invigorate the body and mind.

Winter brings unique challenges for the body, such as coldness, stiffness, fatigue, and a tendency toward lower energy levels. Yoga asanas (postures) can be particularly beneficial in winter as they help warm the body, increase circulation, and improve flexibility. They also support the immune system and combat the physical and mental sluggishness accompanying the colder months. Below are specific yoga asanas for winter, with detailed steps and their advantages.

1. Tadasana (Mountain Pose)

Steps:

Ayurvedic yoga lifestyle for winter

- Stand tall with your feet together or hip-width apart.
- Engage your thighs, lift your kneecaps, and firm your abdomen.
- Stretch your arms overhead with palms facing each other and fingers extended, reaching upward.
- Keep your shoulders relaxed and away from your ears.
- Hold the pose for 20-30 seconds while breathing deeply,
- focusing on your alignment and posture.

Benefits for Winter:

- Increases Energy: Tadasana activates the entire body, creating a sense of alertness and energy, which is helpful when winter fatigue sets in.

Improve Circulation: Improving blood flow is essential in colder weather to prevent stiffness or cold extremities, which can be prevented with the pose.

Posture: Standing tall strengthens the spine and counteracts the tendency to slouch due to cold or lack of movement in winter.

Ayurvedic yoga lifestyle for winter

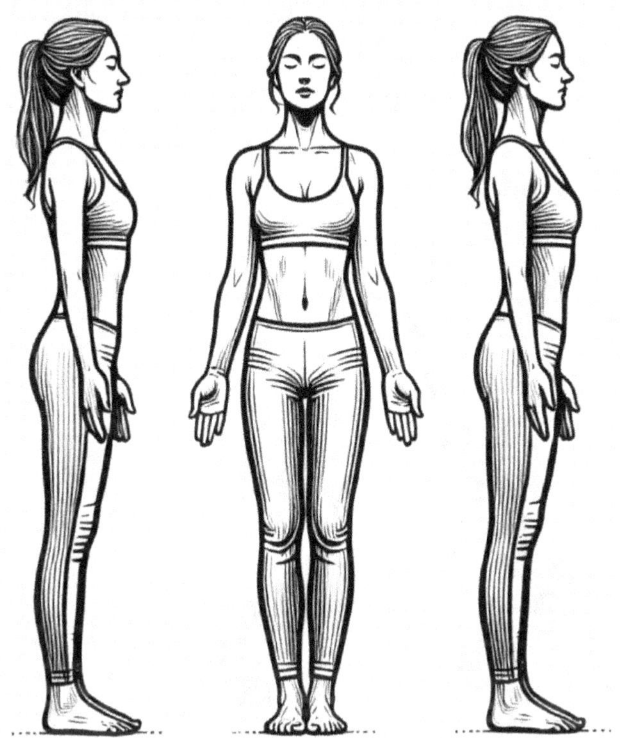

Tadasana (Mountain Pose)

2. Utkatasana (Chair Pose)

Steps:

- Stand with your feet hip-width apart.
- As you inhale, lift your arms above your head, keeping them aligned and parallel.
- Bend your knees as though lowering into an invisible chair, aiming to bring your thighs parallel to the ground.

Ayurvedic yoga lifestyle for winter

- Keep your chest lifted and avoid letting your knees extend beyond your toes.
- Hold the pose for 20-30 seconds, keeping your abdomen engaged and breathing deeply.

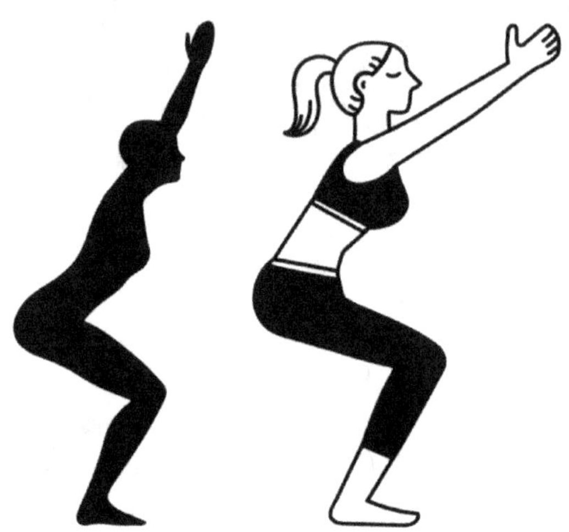

Utkatasana (Chair Pose)

Benefits for Winter:

- Warms the Body: Utkatasana generates internal heat through the strong engagement of leg muscles, helping to combat the cold.
- Strengthens the Legs: This pose strengthens the thighs, calves, and glutes,

Ayurvedic yoga lifestyle for winter

which can become weak from less activity in the winter.

- Stimulates the Circulatory System: The deep bend in the knees helps improve blood flow to the lower body, preventing coldness in the legs and feet

3. Bhujangasana (Cobra Pose)

Steps:

- Lie face down with your legs stretched out and the tops of your feet resting on the mat.
- Position your hands beneath your shoulders, keeping your elbows tucked in close to your sides.
- As you inhale, slowly lift your chest off the ground, extending your arms while keeping a gentle bend in the elbows. Draw your shoulders back and down and look straight ahead or slightly upward.
- Hold this posture for 15 to 30 seconds, breathing deeply throughout.

Ayurvedic yoga lifestyle for winter

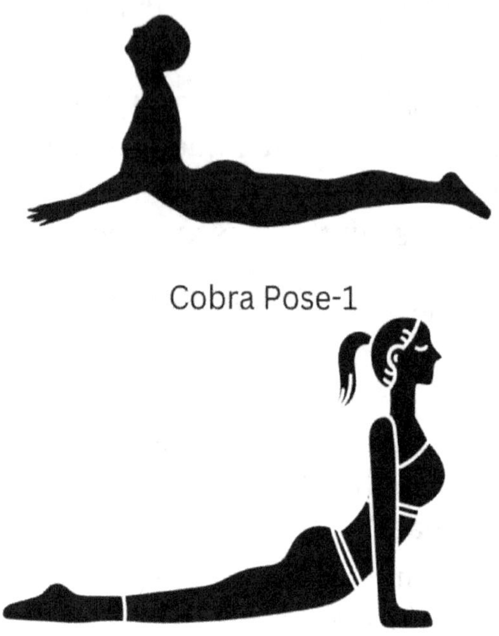

Cobra Pose-1

Cobra Pose-2

Benefits for Winter:

- Warms the Spine: Bhujangasana is excellent for warming the spine and stimulating circulation to the back muscles, which can get stiff in the cold.
- Improves Posture: It counteracts the tendency to hunch or slouch during colder months when we tend to curl up in warm spaces.

Ayurvedic yoga lifestyle for winter

- Opens the Chest: This asana opens the chest and lungs, improving airflow and making it easier to breathe in the dry winter air

4. Setu Bandhasana (Bridge Pose)

Steps:

- Lie on your back with your knees bent and feet flat on the floor, hip-width apart.
- Rest your arms alongside your body, with your palms pressing gently into the floor.
- Press your feet into the floor as you lift your hips up, creating a straight line from your shoulders to your knees.
- Interlace your fingers under your back and roll your shoulders down, lifting your chest toward your chin.
- Hold the position for 20-30 seconds, breathing deeply.

Ayurvedic yoga lifestyle for winter

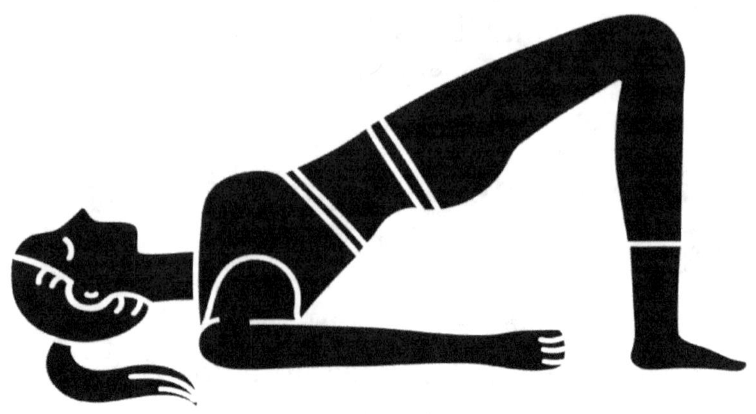

Benefits for Winter:

- Warms the Body: Setu Bandhasana generates warmth by engaging the glutes, thighs, and core muscles, combating winter chill.
- Stimulates the Endocrine System: It activates the thyroid and other endocrine glands, which can help regulate metabolism during the sluggish winter months.
- Relieves Lower Back Pain: It stretches and strengthens the lower back, which can become stiff from sitting indoors more frequently during winter.

Ayurvedic yoga lifestyle for winter

- ## **5.Adho Mukha Svanasana (Downward-Facing Dog)**

Steps:

- Start in a tabletop position with your hands and knees on the floor.
- Tuck your toes and lift your hips toward the ceiling, forming an inverted V shape.
- Place your hands as wide as your shoulders and your feet as wide as your hips.
- Press your heels toward the floor and stretch your arms forward, engaging your core.
- Hold the pose for 30 seconds to one minute, breathing deeply.

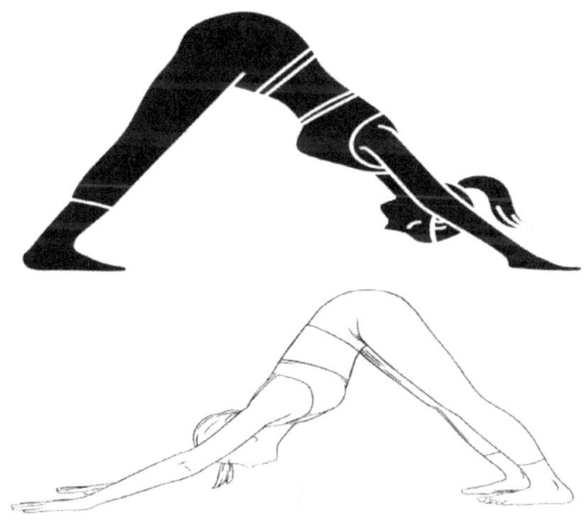

Adho Mukha Svanasana (Downward-Facing Dog)

Ayurvedic yoga lifestyle for winter

Benefits for Winter:

- Increases Circulation: This pose encourages blood flow to the upper body, energizing and warming the body during winter.
- Stretches the Body: It stretches the entire back, hamstrings, calves, and shoulders, preventing stiffness from sitting or hunching.
- Boosts Energy: Downward-Facing Dog is a full-body stretch that helps fight sluggishness by increasing circulation and stimulating the nervous system

6. Virabhadrasana I (Warrior I Pose)

Steps:

- Begin standing with your feet placed wide apart.
- Turn your left foot out 90 degrees and angle your right foot slightly inward.
- Bend your left knee and raise your arms overhead, palms facing each other.
- Square your hips toward the front and sink deeply into the left knee, ensuring it does not extend beyond your ankle.

Ayurvedic yoga lifestyle for winter

- Hold the pose for 20-30 seconds, taking deep breaths.

Benefits for Winter:

- Warms the Body: Warrior I engages large muscle groups, particularly the legs, core, and arms, helping to generate body heat.

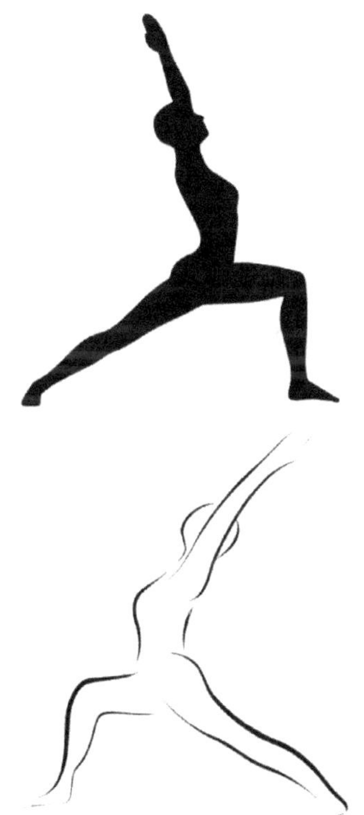

Virabhadrasana I (Warrior I Pose)

Ayurvedic yoga lifestyle for winter

- Improves strength: This pose strengthens the legs, core, and shoulders, enhancing overall physical strength, which is particularly beneficial in the winter months when energy levels may dip.

Opens the Chest: The overhead arms open the chest, encouraging better lung function, especially in dry, cold air

7. Trikonasana (Triangle Pose)

Steps:

- Stand with your feet spread about 3 to 4 feet apart.
- Rotate your right foot 90 degrees outward and slightly turn your left foot inward.
- Stretch your arms out to the sides and then hinge at the waist to reach toward your right leg, placing your right hand on your shin, ankle, or the floor, wherever it is comfortable.
- Keep your left arm pointing toward the ceiling and your gaze either up or toward your left hand.
- Hold the pose for 20-30 seconds, taking deep breaths.

Ayurvedic yoga lifestyle for winter

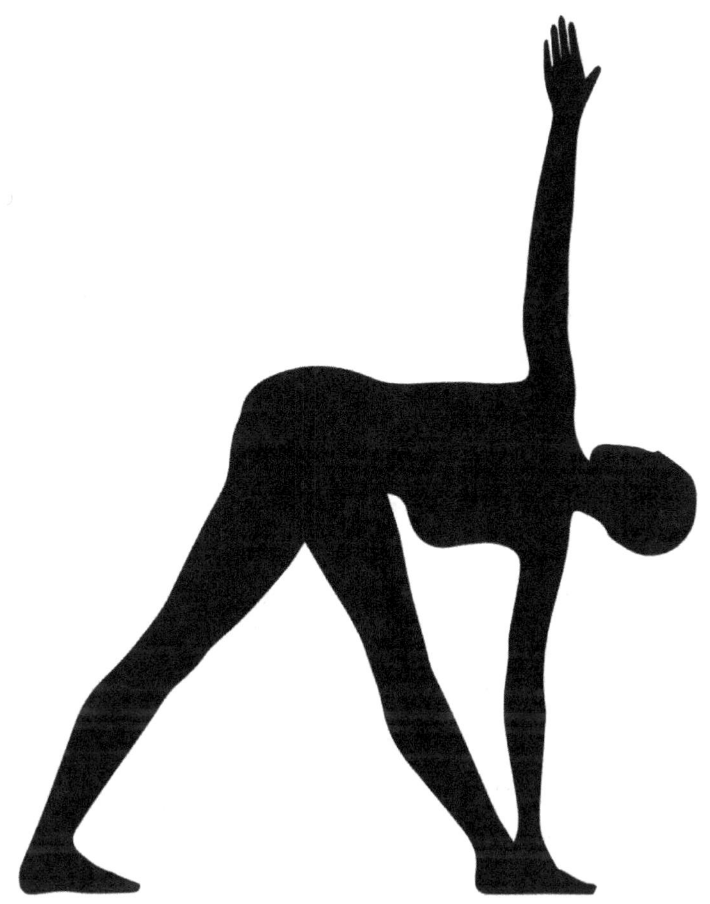

Trikonasana (Triangle Pose)

Benefits for Winter:

- Improves Flexibility: This asana increases flexibility in the hips, hamstrings, and spine, helping to prevent the stiffness that often occurs in cold weather.

Ayurvedic yoga lifestyle for winter

- Stimulates the Digestive System: Triangle pose encourages better digestion by twisting the torso, which can be beneficial during winter when the digestive system tends to slow down.
- Opens the Chest: It also helps to open the chest and improve lung capacity, which is helpful when breathing in dry or cold air

8. Supta Baddha Konasana

(Reclining Bound Angle Pose)

Steps:

- Lie down on your back, bringing the soles of your feet together and allowing your knees to fall out to the sides.
- Place your hands on your abdomen or extend them out to the sides with palms facing up.
- Relax your body and take deep, slow breaths, allowing the chest and hips to open naturally.

Ayurvedic yoga lifestyle for winter

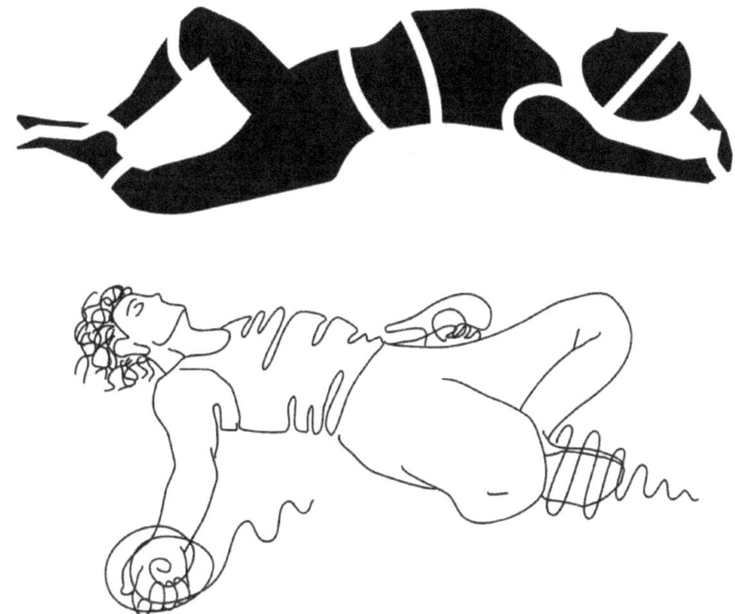

- Stay in this position for 1-3 minutes, breathing deeply.

Benefits for Winter:

- Calms the Nervous System: This restorative pose helps soothe the body and mind, reducing any stress or anxiety that may arise during the winter months.

Ayurvedic yoga lifestyle for winter

- Opens the Hips: It releases tension in the hips and groin, which can become tight from being indoors and sedentary.
- Promotes Relaxation: It promotes deep relaxation, making it a great pose to practice at the end of a winter yoga session to calm the body and prepare for sleep.
- reducing any stress or anxiety that may arise during winter.
- Opens the Hips: It releases tension in the hips and groin, which can become tight from being indoors and sedentary.
- Promotes Relaxation: It promotes deep relaxation, making it a great pose to practice at the end of a winter yoga session to calm the body and prepare for sleep.

10.Salamba Sarvangasana (Shoulder Stand)

Steps:

- Lie on your back and lift your legs straight up, bringing them over your head.
- Support your back with your hands, and lift your hips toward the ceiling, keeping your legs straight.

Ayurvedic yoga lifestyle for winter

- Ensure your neck and spine are aligned and your gaze is directed toward your chest.

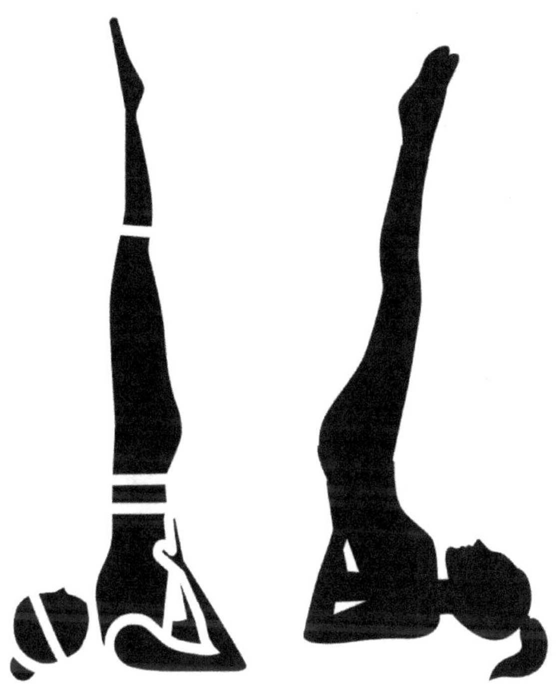

Salamba Sarvangasana (Shoulder Stand)

- Hold the pose for 20-30 seconds to 1 minute, breathing deeply.

Benefits for Winter:

Ayurvedic yoga lifestyle for winter

- Increase Circulation: The inversion improves circulation,
- helping to prevent cold feet or hands.
- Strengthens the Upper Body: It strengthens the arms, shoulders, and core, which can help combat the sedentary nature of winter.

  Calms the Mind: This inversion is great for calming the nervous system and can help alleviate winter-related stress or depression

Ayurvedic yoga lifestyle for winter

WRAPPING UP

This book provides a brief yet insightful guide to navigating the winter season with the timeless wisdom of Ayurveda and Yoga.

In winter, Kapha and Vata doshas interplay can lead to lymphatic stagnation, dryness, and weakened immunity. Ayurveda addresses these challenges through warm, hydrating, and nourishing practices that counteract doshic imbalances. Maintaining a balanced diet, engaging in regular movement, and using supportive Ayurvedic remedies, the lymphatic system (Rasa Dhatu) can remain healthy and robust, ensuring efficient detoxification and immune function throughout the season.

Embrace the essence of winter and celebrate its unique beauty through yoga. During this season, our bodies and minds often feel sluggish, stiff, and cold. The yoga asanas outlined in this book- such as Tadasana, Utkatasana, Bhujangasana, Setu Bandhasana, Adho Mukha Svanasana, Virabhadrasana I, Trikonasana, Supta Baddha Konasana, and Salamba Sarvangasana, are thoughtfully designed to warm the body, invigorate the mind, and cultivate inner vitality.

Additionally, following a structured daily routine (Dinacharya) helps pacify Vata's erratic nature and stabilise Kapha. Adequate sleep is crucial during this season, allowing the lymphatic system to regenerate and function optimally.

Ayurveda and Yoga empower us to manage our lives more efficiently.

Ayurvedic yoga lifestyle for winter

A healthy body and mind enable us to navigate the demands of our busy lifestyles with greater ease and resilience. This e-book explores fundamental practices for managing our lifestyle and aligning ourselves with the land's geography and seasonal changes, all while minimising harm to the earth.

By staying mindful of these practices, we can maintain our health and vitality, something we often overlook in our fast-paced lives; we must also remember that we are cohabitants on this planet, sharing space with nature and its intricate elements. Respecting the balance of the world's natural systems is not just a choice but a necessity. Ignoring this balance leads to health and environmental crises, as exemplified by the global challenges of climate change and warming. Unhealthy individuals create an unhealthy world.

True wellness begins from within each of us.

Take care of your health, nurture your connection with nature, and enjoy the beauty of winter. May this e-book gently remind you to cherish your well-being and the world around you

Ayurvedic yoga lifestyle for winter

IMPORTANT NOTE

This Book focuses on the advantages of Ayurveda and yoga for maintaining well-being and health during winter. The pranayama and yoga asanas included in this Book are specifically tailored to address winter needs. For a deeper exploration, we recommend checking our books dedicated to pranayama, meditation, and winter-specific yoga practices, as these are comprehensive subjects.

If you are a beginner in yoga and pranayama, we encourage you to refer to our beginner-friendly Books for detailed guidance and structured programs tailored to your level.

Ayurvedic yoga lifestyle for winter

RESOURCES

Ashtanga Hrudaya Sutrasthana

Adishivyoga - Reference Note, Class Note

'Heal with the Wisdom of Nature, Live with the Power of Ayurveda.'

Ayurvedic yoga lifestyle for winter

AFTERWORD

In today's fast-paced world, it's easy to become disconnected from nature, forgetting that we are a part of it. This separation contributes to many challenges we now face, seasonal changes, stress, and the rise of new diseases. Reconnecting with the natural environment, aligning with the weather and geography around us, has never been more essential.

Many people ask, "How is it possible to live in harmony with nature when life is already so busy?" The good news is that it *is* possible. This guide was created to support that very journey toward health, balance, and awareness.

Drawing on timeless principles from Ayurveda and Yoga, this book offers practical, holistic tools that have stood the test for centuries. These ancient systems help illuminate a path toward well-being that is sustainable and rooted in nature.

Experience in health education and counselling has shown that much illness stems from a lack of knowledge about life, the body, and the impacts of modern lifestyles. Culture plays a significant role in shaping daily habits, and while not all cultural norms promote health, there is wisdom to be found across traditions. By thoughtfully adopting supportive practices from

Ayurvedic yoga lifestyle for winter

different cultures, we can take proactive steps to protect and enhance our health.

As the adage reminds us, "Prevention is better than a cure." This guide distils over three decades of accumulated insights, study, and lived experience into a concise resource designed to help navigate the seasons with ease and awareness.

The aim is simple: to provide accessible, effective guidance that can be easily woven into everyday routines. May this book inspire a more harmonious way of living, one that listens to the rhythms of nature and honours the interconnectedness of life.

Ayurvedic yoga lifestyle for winter

ABOUT THE AUTHOR

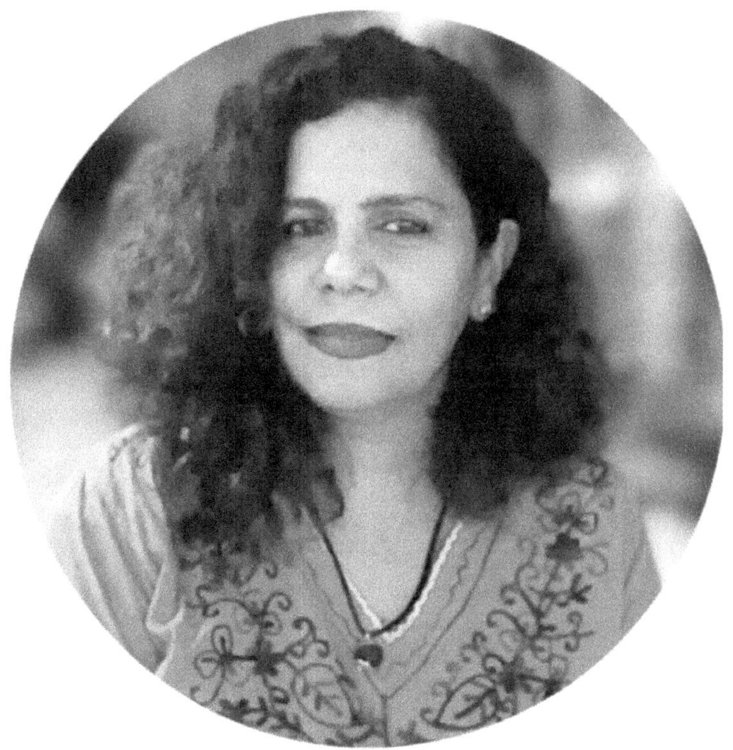

S. Panikkal

As a qualified Ayurveda Wellness Counsellor, Psychologist, and Yoga Therapy educator, I've dedicated my work to guiding individuals toward mental, physical, and spiritual health. Being of Indian origin and living in Switzerland, I've had the unique opportunity to work with people from diverse cultures, races, and religions, enriching my understanding and approach to holistic wellness.

Ayurvedic yoga lifestyle for winter

Every day, I strive to contribute to a mentally and physically fit world, helping People connect with themselves and live their best lives. Through this book,

I hope to share some of the knowledge and insights I've gained along the way, and I look forward to being a part of your journey to a healthier and more fulfilling life.

https://sharmilasbooks.com/about

https://www.instagram.com/rewire_ur_brain

https://sharmilapds.blogspot.com

Ayurvedic yoga lifestyle for winter